Building Up

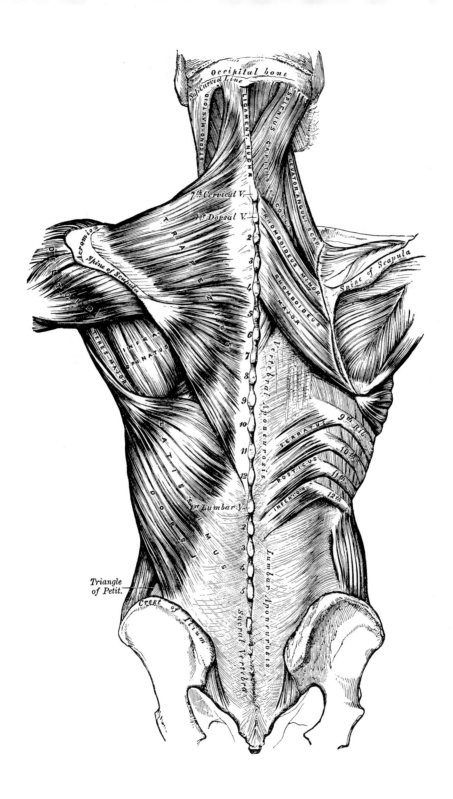

THE YOUNG ATHLETE'S GUIDE TO WEIGHT TRAINING

Building Up

PETE BROCCOLETTI

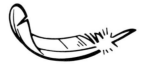

ICARUS PRESS

South Bend, Indiana

1981

Building Up
copyright© 1981 by Pete Broccoletti

Principal photographer for exercises was James Cordean.

Icarus Press, Inc.
Post Office Box 1225
South Bend, Indiana 46624

Library of Congress Cataloging in Publication Data

Broccoletti, Peter Paul Lusardi.
   Building up.

   Includes index.
   1. Weight lifting. 2. Physical education
and training. 3. Exercise. I. Title.
GV546.5.B76   613.7'1   81-6582
ISBN 0-89651-053-0   AACR2
ISBN 0-89651-054-9 (pbk.)

Thanks go to Rafael Guerrero
for the use of his Gold Coast Gym in Ft. Lauderdale
and his young members who have appeared herein as models:
Chris Duffy, Jeff Fee, Greg Wright, Ty Thornton, and Rocky Lee.
Thanks also go to George Smith, head football coach at
St. Thomas Aquinas High School in Ft. Lauderdale
for the use of his school facilities and supplying me
with the following fine young high school students as models:
Joe Walsh, Fred Rohwedder, Paul Corley, and Mike Higgins.
Without George's and Rafael's assistance,
I would not have been able to complete this book.
Their advice and encouragement have been appreciated,
and they are certainly a credit to their professions.

CONTENTS

INTRODUCTION

While traveling around the country these last few years giving weight-training clinics at the high-school level, I have had numerous requests for a weight-training book specifically for boys aged 12 to 17. Models in my previous books (*The Notre Dame Weight-Training Program for Football, The Notre Dame Weight-Training Program for Baseball, Hockey, Wrestling & Your Body,* and *Shape Up for Soccer*) were college students; some even became professional athletes. And the routines in those books were vigorous. But this book is designed for a younger athlete.

A boy in his early teens is going through great physiological changes and growing at his greatest rate. He needs all the rest and food he can get (within reason) to help him grow to his fullest potential. He needs to rest up for school, sports, and other activities. Therefore, the young man needs a less rigorous weight program than a man needs.

In this book I have redone the exercises using high-school student models that the 12-to 17-year old can relate to but ones that look good enough that he would want to emulate. I have devised a nutrition chapter that should be easy to understand and appealing. The sports I have included in this book are the most popular team sports for youth, and since many athletes participate in more than one sport during the school year, breaking the routine schedule into off-season and in-season programs (as I have done in my other books) might not be appropriate here. Therefore, I have placed asterisks in the routines sections to indicate those exercises meant as maintenance ones to be done *during* the season but which can also be performed as *transitions* from one sport to another. So if the reader is playing football but will later be playing basketball, he would do the exercises marked by asterisks in the football routine. Then, when basketball season comes along, he would do the basketball exercises marked there by asterisks.

This is slightly different from the normal procedure at the college or pro level of sports. At that level, we use the off-season to build strength or size and then use the in-season for maintenance of that size and strength. But by performing these basic exercises two or three times a week during the season, the young athlete will be able to build size, strength, and endurance. It is important to remember, though, that a young athlete should not work out the day before a game, for his muscles will not be restored enough by game time to enable him to play his best.

I am sure that following these routines will help such an athlete not only to grow bigger and stronger but will help him play better and with less injury. For those that have not been lifting weights, I recommend participating in calisthenics for three to six months (depending upon one's physical condition), prior to beginning a weight-training program. Calisthenics such as push-ups, sit-ups, and leg raises are good to get the body ready for the rigorous training ahead.

For those with any physical problems, consult with a doctor before beginning weight training. An ounce of prevention is important because it is easy to aggravate an injury.

NUTRITION

Nutrition is one of the most important things in your life right now. It is more important to you right now than even to the professional athletes because you are going through the greatest rate of physical growth in your life; the pro has grown just about all he is going to do. You could lift weights two hours a day, six days a week, and not notice significant growth if you were not on a proper diet.

A young athlete needs more than 3,000 calories a day from well-balanced meals to function properly and grow. The demands on your body — playing football, basketball, and other sports in addition to weight training — are great.

Protein

The essentials that our bodies need are proteins, fats, carbohydrates, mineral salts, vitamins, and water. Protein is essential because it is the body's primary building material and is the basis of living cells. Besides your muscles, your skin, hair, nails, eyes, brain, and organs are composed of protein. Protein makes up antibodies, our body's defense mechanisms.

When you lift weights vigorously, you break down muscle tissues, which process is called *catabolism*. When you rest and take in enough protein, your muscles are repaired by the process of *anabolism*. But to grow bigger and stronger, anabolism must be greater than catabolism.

The best sources of protein are milk and eggs, fish and meat. These contain all the eight essential amino acids, which are the building blocks

Unfortunately, most vitamins and minerals are boiled or fried out of the food at institutions. In these instances, I recommend either a strong multiple vitamin and mineral each day or one 500-milligram vitamin C; one B complex of 25-gram strength; one vitamin E, 400 I.U., and one mineral compound each day. But again, I stress that you generally do not need these supplements if you are eating three home-cooked, balanced meals a day.

The following is a list of important vitamins and minerals:

Vitamin A	important for eyesight as well as normal cell growth, healthy skin, and skeletal development.
B Complex	important as a whole for energy production, to combat stress and for nail and skin maintenance, digestive juice secretions, blood vessels and eye maintenance.
Vitamin B 15	not a vitamin as determined by the FDA but a food supplement. It is supposed to be effective in treating circulatory disorders, preventive aging and heart disease and helping stamina.
Vitamin C	(ascorbic acid) prevents scurvy, aids in the formation of collagen, which holds all cells together. It also builds up the resistance to shock and infection. Dr. Linus Pauling claims that megadoses of C help prevent colds.
Vitamin D	necessary for growth of bones and teeth and prevents fatigue. It is found easiest in milk and eggs.
Vitamin E	still the subject of a lot of research but aids in supplying oxygen to the cells.
Minerals	Calcium, phosphorus, magnesium, sodium, potassium, sulfur, chlorine, iron, copper, cobalt, iodine, manganese, zinc, and flourine are needed in

your daily diet. Because these are found in most foods and a deficiency is not as likely as a vitamin deficiency, I will not go into detail with them. Remember, your sweat is just not water but contains minerals that are commonly called electrolytes — potassium, magnesium, and sodium. Based on this premise, a number of companies have come out with drinks to replace these lost electrolytes. There is some question whether they are of much use other than quenching thirst and replacing lost fluids because of the time it takes for the minerals to do their job. Another important need is for potassium. A few years ago, a number of people who went on a liquid protein diet died because their diet lacked potassium. A banana or tomato each day will supply you with all the potassium your body needs.

Eat fresh fruits and vegetables. Processing and packaging of canned fruits and vegetables take too much of the minerals and vitamins out. I also recommend that you avoid white bread because the flour is too processed. Eat French, Italian, whole wheat, rye, or pumpernickel bread. Also, I recommend avoiding refined sugar because it is bad for you and can cause depression when you come down from the sugar high.

Your Diet

If you are trying to gain weight, I recommend snacks such as yogurt laced with wheat germ or brewer's yeast, sardines on wheat thins, peanut butter sandwiches on whole wheat bread, or just unsalted dry peanuts. For those who are finding it hard to get bigger, I recommend a protein drink, preferably a milk-and-egg protein drink.

of protein. Of the twenty-two different amino acids known and needed in forming tissues, all but eight are manufactured in the human body. Therefore, the essential eight amino acids must be supplied in our food.

The National Resources Council recommends 0.42 grams of protein per pound of body weight. I think that if you eat 1/2 gram of protein per pound of body weight, you will be all right. Any excess protein is just excreted out.

Besides milk and eggs, which I think are the most important things you can be eating, I rate next in order of preference, fish (especially tuna), liver, chicken, then steak and roast beef. Broiled fish is great because it is high in protein and low in fat and calories.

Do not worry about cholesterol in eggs. First of all, you are too young to be worrying about that and, second, there is lecithin in eggs, which is a homogenizing agent and breaks down fat and cholesterol into miniscule particles that can pass readily into the tissue. You should be eating four eggs and drinking at least one quart of milk a day.

Fats

Fats are necessary for the maintenance of good health and form part of every cell. They permit important intestinal bacteria to multiply, are needed for sex and adrenal hormones, help water balance, transport vitamins A, D, E, and K to the cells, and act as a homogenizing agent. The foods that are high in essential fatty acids are French dressing, salad oils, avacados, nuts, and mayonnaise.

Carbohydrates

Carbohydrates, when ingested, break down quickly into glucose, which is simple sugar, and is used almost immediately as a supply of energy. They are best obtained through fruits and vegetables. Generally you need one-half gram of carbohydrate for each pound of bodyweight, but pick your carbs from good sources and avoid junk food like cake, cookies, candies, and soda. Many people go on a high protein diet, with a low amount of carbs kept on their diet for energy. The people that tried to go on a zero carb diet found they had no energy.

Water and Fiber

Water is important to the athlete because our muscles and bodies are made up of mostly water. It is best to drink spring water that has not had additives and is rich in natural minerals. Drinking plenty of water also flushes out your system of the poisons in certain foods, and the water is needed in perspiration so that the body may cleanse itself from within and keep your temperature down.

Fiber, nature's laxative, is the nondigestable part of food in whole grains, nuts, fresh fruits, and vegetables. It is a necessary part of your diet. An interesting fact is that cultures that stick to high-fiber diets do not have a high incidence of digestive problems.

Vitamins & Minerals

Vitamins are necessary for good health, and the young athlete needs more than the average person. His body store of vital nutrients is being constantly depleted through his great amount of physical exercise. I think that generally a boy who eats three big home-cooked meals a day and nutritional snacks, such as yogurt or nuts, gets all the vitamins and minerals he needs. Vitamin deficiencies occur when he is not eating all his meals, especially at an institution like a live-in prep school. Unfortunately, most vitamins and minerals are boiled or fried out of the food at institutions. In these instances, I recommend either a strong multiple vitamin and mineral each day or one 500-milligram vitamin C; one B complex of 25-gram strength; one vitamin E, 400 I.U., and one mineral compound each day. But again, I stress that you generally do not need these supplements if you are eating three home-cooked, balanced meals a day.

The following are some weight-training recipes:

Pineapple Delight: ¼ cut-up pineapple, 6 oz. cottage cheese, 1 oz. wheat germ, 3 oz. cream, and a few ice cubes. Blend in a blender and drink it down.

Fruit Drink Pleasures: 1 cup unsweetened pineapple juice, 1 cup coconut milk, 2 tablespoons protein powder, 1 tablespoon wheat germ oil. Mix in blender.

Banana Surprise: 1 banana, 1 cup milk, 1 cup unsweetened pineapple juice, 2 tablespoons wheat germ, ¼ papaya. Mix in blender.

Protein Snack: 6 oz. cottage cheese, 6 oz. plain yogurt, and ¼ pineapple. Mix in blender.

Papaya Delights: ¼ pineapple, 6 oz. plain yogurt, 2 tablespoons protein supplement, and 6 oz. coconut milk. Mix in blender.

Strawberry Delight: 6 oz. whipping cream, 10 strawberries, 2 tablespoons of wheat germ, 1 piece of papaya. Blend and let freeze for four hours.

Remember if you want to get bigger, you are going to have to eat more. More protein and exercise builds bigger muscles. Your most important meal is breakfast. Get up early and pile those eggs on those pancakes. When you eat dinner, do not eat one piece of chicken, but three or four. Avoid junk food. Make sure you get plenty of sleep. Your body needs that time to recuperate, to build back up. Most of you need at least eight hours of sleep each day. Do not eat during the two hours before you work out except for a piece of fruit or drink. Blood is necessary in the stomach for digestion to take place, and muscle exertion will steal blood away from the digestion process, making it difficult to digest food properly. This can lead to stomach cramps and nausea. It is all right to sip liquids as you work out.

Steroids

Steroids are the last subject in this chapter because I want my comments on this chapter to remain fresh in your mind. Although a significant number of bodybuilders and a number of other athletes have used them, I am definitely opposed to them. Not just because they are not natural or because you shrink quickly after usage is stopped. The dangerous side effects that might occur are liver and kidney damage, impotency, skin problems or loss of hair. Since they have not been around long, there has not been time enough to check for possible damages to human chromosomes. The children of those who took steroids might be born with birth defects. The 1980s will bring a lot of answers to many questions about the dangers of steroids.

In summary, I always recommend that my trainees avoid steroids as well as any other drugs.

PART I:

EXERCISES
BY BODY PART

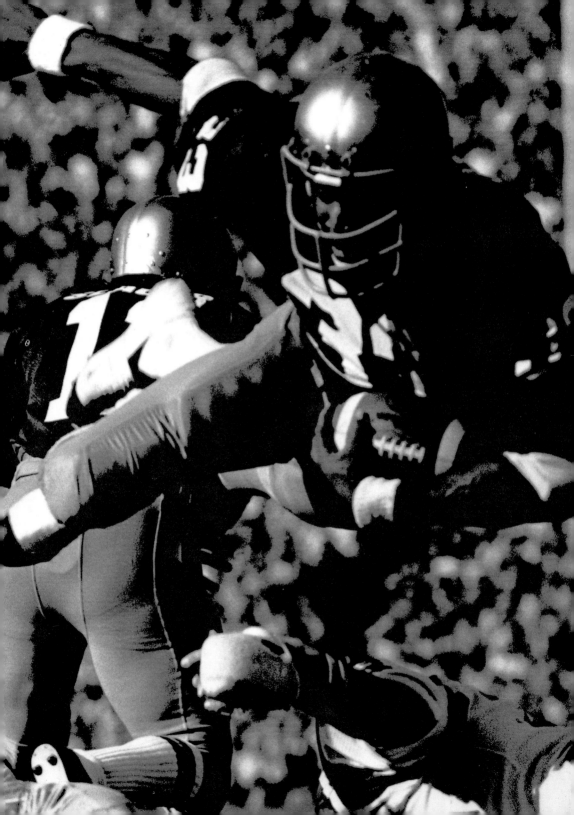

FLEXIBILITY

Thank God the old wives' tale that weight lifters are musclebound and cannot play sports is being put to rest. Does Walter Payton of the Chicago Bears or basketball star Adrian Dantley look inflexible? They do not, and they are regular weight trainers. Carl Yastrzemski of the Boston Red Sox is another weight-trained athlete.

The negative aspect of each weight-lifting exercise stretches the muscles and promotes flexibility. Even so, a special flexibility program is crucial. Stretching is important to promote flexibility, for warming up, cooling down, and preventing injuries. When you lift weights, you are contracting the muscles; so to promote optimum flexibility, you need to stretch out, which elongates your muscles.

Athletes have to be flexible both to prevent injuries and to reach the limit of their athletic potential. In football, being flexible helps prevent muscle tears and allows you to make that cut to spring lose for a long run, to make that clutch catch, or to avoid a blocker. In basketball, flexibility promotes rebounding and allows you to stay with the man you are guarding. In baseball, it means being able to dive and make that difficult catch. Soccer players need to be flexible not only to prevent muscle tears but to be able to get their legs out far enough to kick the ball or to stretch out to tackle. The need for flexibility in the swimmer is obvious. In wrestling, flexibility could make the difference in being taken down and pinned. And for general fitness enthusiasts, flexibility is important for injury prevention and general health.

Some teams stretch out for six minutes before practicing or lifting, but I think a good three or four minutes of stretching is sufficient inside where it is warmer. Obviously, outside on a cold day you will need more stretching to prepare for the contest. I also recommend stretching out after your workout as a cool-down. Just as it is important to warm up to prepare your body for what is to come, it is important to cool down after working out. Your body has been revved up, and you just do not want to shut it off completely and at once.

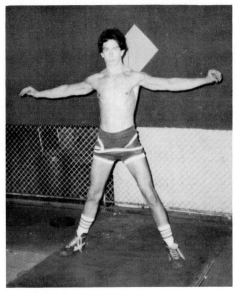

A1: Circular Shoulder Rotation
From this starting position, rotate the neck in a full circle, extending the head as far back as it will go. Use the same motion for the arms and trunk, completing at least 10 full circles. These exercises will loosen up the key muscle groups.

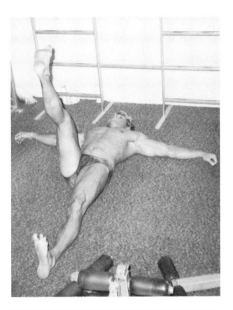

B1-2: Hamstring Trunk Rotation
This should be done with both legs straight and your hands on the ground. Attempt to touch your right foot to the left hand and the left foot to the right hand. Stretch the hamstrings 2 to 3 times in this manner.

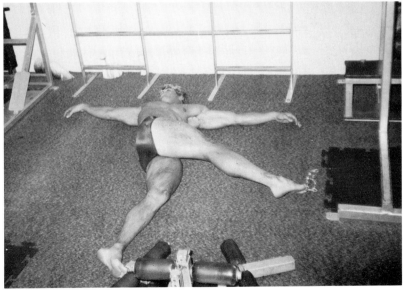

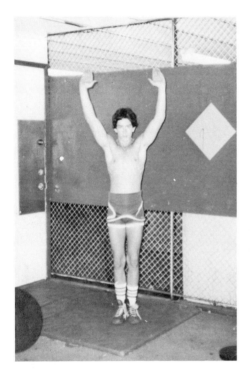

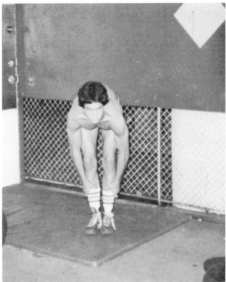

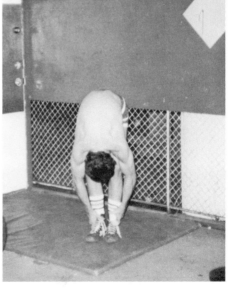

C1-3: Hamstring Stretch I *(left)*
This exercise will properly loosen up the hamstring muscle, which together with the quadriceps provide 80 percent of the knee's support. With hands fully extended into the air, bend over, being careful not to bend your knees. The motion should be a smooth movement. Be careful not to jerk down and pull the hamstring. Grasp your ankles and continue the motion until your head touches your knees.

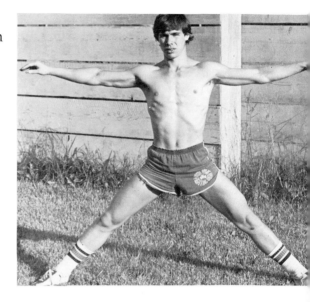

D1-2: Hamstring Stretch II
Start in a position such as the one used in shoulder, neck, and trunk circles but this time spread the legs as far apart as possible. Grasp the ankle with both hands and attempt to touch your chin to the knee. Repeat with both legs 2 to 3 times.

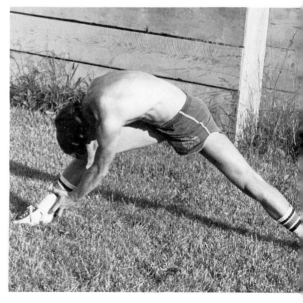

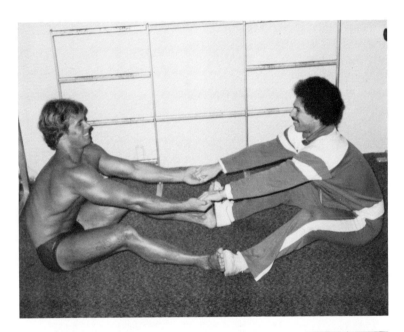

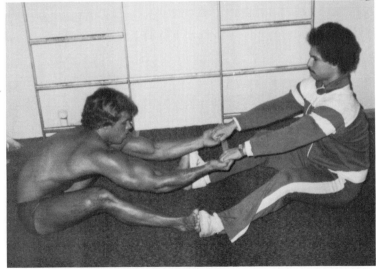

E1-2: Partner Stretch
With your partner facing you, stretch open the legs until your feet touch the inside of his ankles. While grasping each other's wrists, pull back while your partner offers resistance. Repeat the exercise with reversed roles.

F1: Flip-Over Hamstring Stretch
Lying flat on the ground with your hands at your side, lock the knees and spread your legs as far apart as possible. Raise your legs until your toes touch the ground. Those suffering from lower-back problems should avoid this exercise.

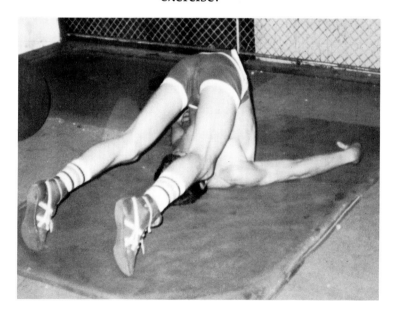

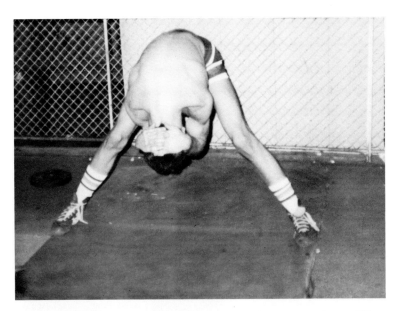

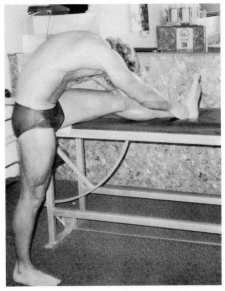

G1: Bent-Over Hamstring Stretch *(above)*

Starting in the spread-eagled position, place your hands behind your head and attempt to touch the ground with your head. Stretch slowly and avoid jerking.

H1: Hamstring Groin Stretch I

Place your leg at a right-angled position and grasp the ankle of the horizontal leg while attempting to touch your chin to your knee.

I1: Hamstring Groin Stretch II
Starting in the same position as
the previous exercise, grasp the
ankle of the standing leg and
touch the chin to the knee while
keeping your knees straight.

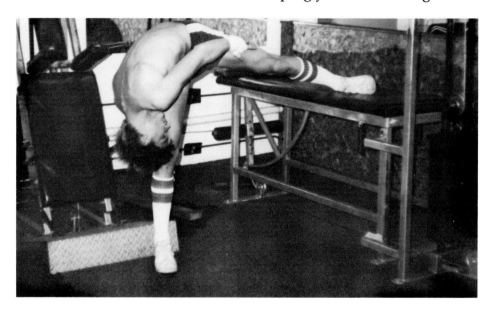

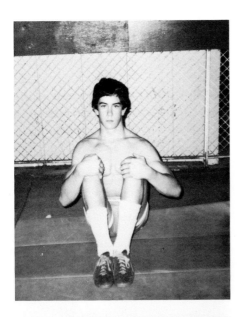

J1-2: Lotus Groin Stretch

Start in the lotus position with ankles together and hands on knees. Push down on the knees and try to touch the ground.

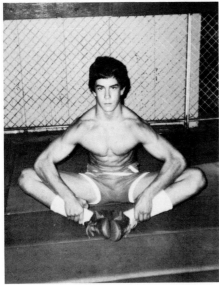

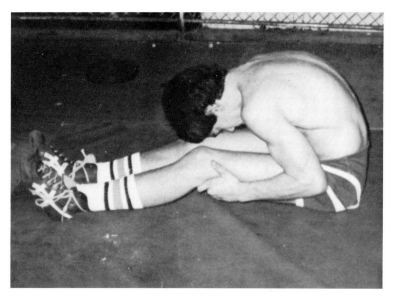

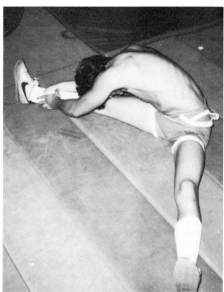

K1: Hamstring Lower-Back Stretch (*above*)
Beginning in a sitting position, grasp behind the calf and try to touch your forehead to your knees. Be careful not to bounce down, but rather do it in one easy motion to maximize the benefit to the hamstring and lower back.

L1: Modified Hurdler's Stretch
With both legs spread apart, keep the knee touching the ground and then attempt to touch your forehead to your knee.

M1: Hurdler's Stretch
Change your position slightly
from the previous exercise by
bending one knee while keeping
the legs apart at a right angle.
Stretch the hamstrings by
leaning forward on your straight
leg while you try to keep the
knee touching the ground to
stretch the quadriceps.

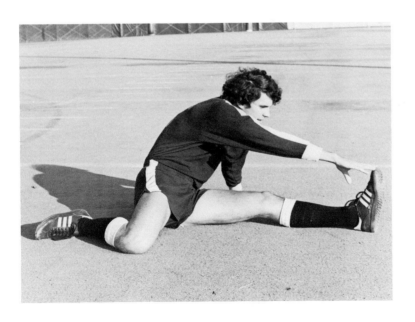

N1: Negative Dip

This is the finest stretching exercise for upper-body flexibility. Just raise yourself up on the dipping bar and then let yourself down slowly, doing the negative aspect of the dip only.

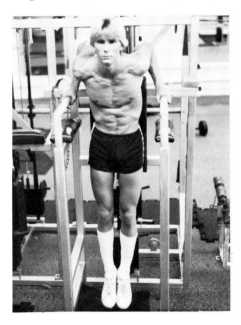

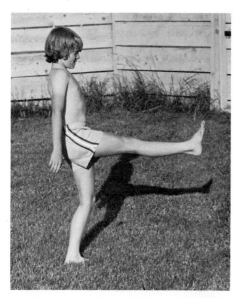

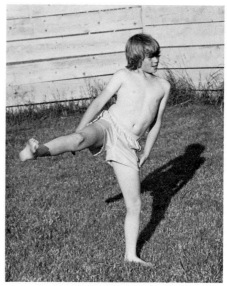

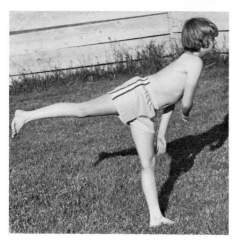

O1-3: Leg Extension
Extend the leg while keeping it as straight as possible in several different directions. You may need some help from a partner to get the full extension in some instances.

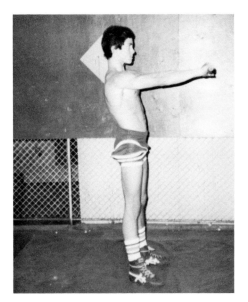 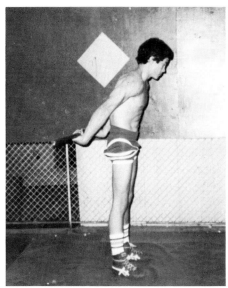

P1-2: Bar Stretch
Hold a bar or bat at the ends in
front of you at shoulder height.
Extend the bar slowly over your
head and down to waist level.

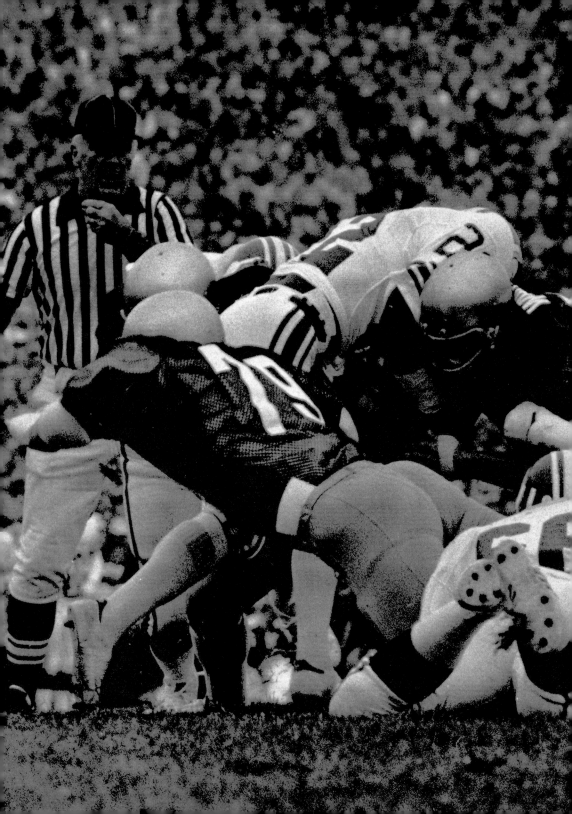

DELTOIDS

"Shoulders make the man" is often heard, and it is very true, since broad shoulders can make a man stand out. Heredity plays the largest part in determining how big you will be, but weight lifting can help develop you to the optimum. The endomorph is the chubby type of person, the ectomorph the tall and skinny person, and the mesomorph the natural athletic build. Although it will be easier for the mesomorph type of person to develop big shoulders, the chubby and the tall, skinny type can also, but it will take more work.

The deltoid has three heads to it — the anterior (front head), the lateral (side head), and the posterior (rear head). The front head is most easily built up because it is worked in any pressing movement. The lateral head is a little harder to develop but responds well to lateral raises. These parts of your deltoids are the part that makes you look broader. Although the posterior (rear) head is the most difficult to build up and usually is the most neglected, it can be developed with behind-the-neck presses, bent-over lateral raises, and behind-the-neck chin-ups.

Deltoids are crucial in football. You need them built up to prevent injuries, principally shoulder separations, which are so common in football. Your shoulders are more dependent on the supporting muscles than any other part of your body. In football, your shoulders are used in blocking, tackling, in absorbing and giving punishment. Quarterbacks would suffer fewer shoulder injuries when they get sacked if they built up their deltoids. You also use your deltoids in passing.

In basketball, your deltoids come into play in defense, holding your arms up, fighting for a rebound, and in your shot.

In baseball, your deltoids are used in hitting and throwing. Shoulder power can make the difference between a home run and a single. Sore shoulders are a common complaint among baseball players but can be prevented by developing those deltoids.

Soccer players have also been known to suffer shoulder injuries, which might have been prevented by weight training. Collisions are not uncommon in soccer! The goalie especially needs this work.

No matter which swimming event you enter, strong shoulders will be of prime importance. A swimmer without broad muscular shoulders is almost unthinkable. Wrestlers are another group that suffer shoulder injuries and therefore it is crucial for wrestlers to build up their shoulders. The deltoids are also used in takedowns, reversals, control, and defense. You also need strong deltoids in your moves such as overhooking, switching, recovering to all fours from the breakdown and in initiating standups.

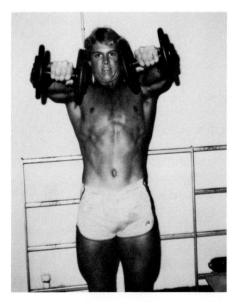

A1: Front Deltoid Raise

These deltoid raises are designed to develop the anterior deltoids. Start in a standing position and grip the dumbbells, using a palms-down technique. Raise the dumbbells until they are even with the shoulders and then continue to raise them directly overhead. Be careful not to bend your elbows while performing this exercise so as not to take away from the usefulness of the movement.

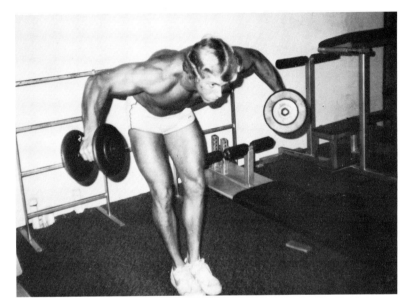

B1: Bent-Over Lateral Raise
The posterior deltoids will be the
object of this exercise. Bend over
until your back is parallel to the
floor. Use a palms-down grip to
lift the dumbbells until they are
even with your shoulders.
Conclude the movement by
slowly lowering the dumbbells
back to their starting position.
Standing lateral raises can also be
accomplished for the lateral
deltoids by performing the
exercise in the same manner,
starting in a standing position.

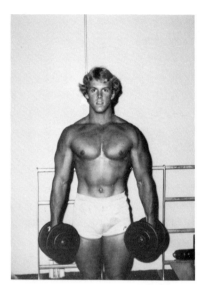 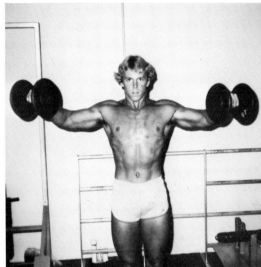

C1-2: Standing Lateral Raise

Stand up with your arms extended downward and with your palms facing each other. Raise the dumbbells to your side and above your shoulders. This exercise does a good job of pumping the lateral, or side, head of your deltoids.

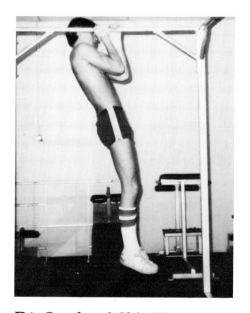

D1: Overhand Chin-Up

This chin-up develops all three heads of the deltoids. Grip the bar with an overhand grip, standing sideways beneath the bar. Pull yourself up until your chin touches the bar and then repeat the chin-up — this time bringing your head up on the opposite side of the bar.

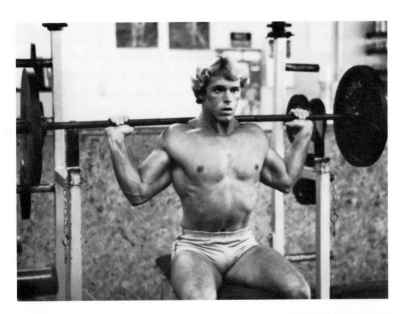

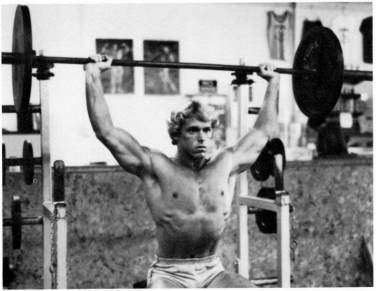

E1-2: Seated, Behind-the-Neck Military Press

The deltoids and triceps are the target of the sitting military press. From the seated position, rest the barbell on the back of your shoulders. Press the barbell upwards, remembering to exhale as you begin your press.

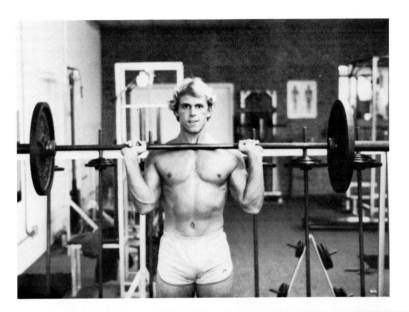

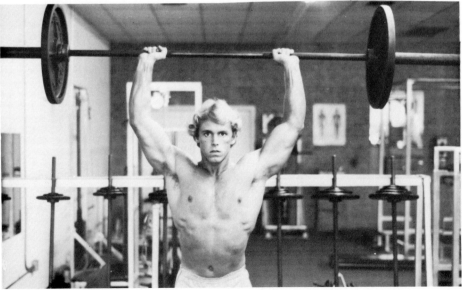

F1-2: Standing Military Press

This variation is similar to the seated press, but can be done from a position on the front or back of the shoulders. Use a shoulder-width grip and proceed to clean the barbell as you normally would. Then press straight up from the position in front of your shoulders. For the behind-the-back military press, clean the bar to the front of your shoulders and then boost it over your head and onto the back of your shoulders. Perform the rest of the exercise as you would any other press.

G1-2: Standing Dumbbell Press

You may do this exercise either alternately or both together. While standing straight and holding a dumbbell on your shoulder, press straight over your head. Do not jerk or bounce the dumbbell off your shoulder.

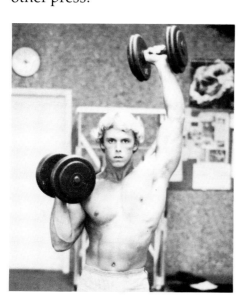

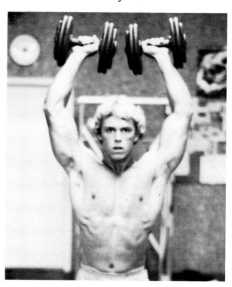

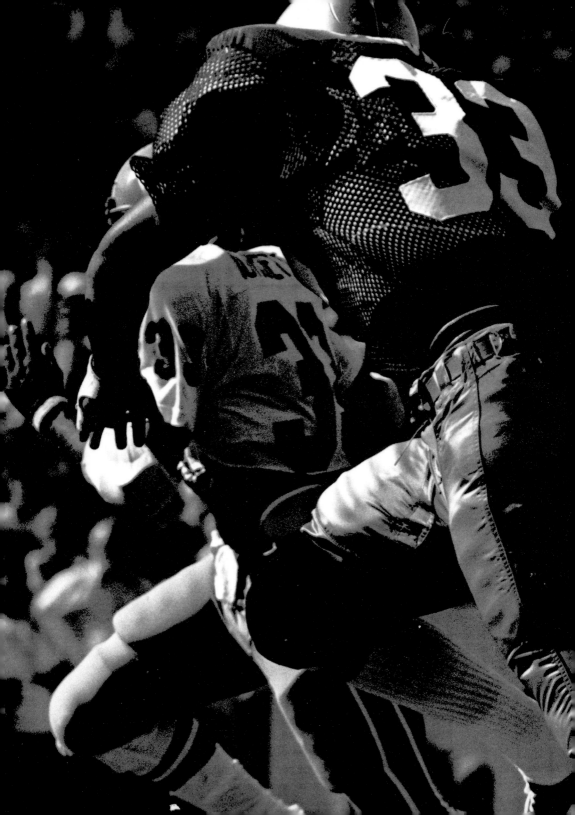

BACK

The largest single muscle group in the back is the latissimus dorsi (lats). Lats need to be worked at every angle to develop the wide, inside, and middle parts. The wide V-look is developed by lat pulldowns and wide-grip chin-ups. To develop the inside you do narrow-grip lat pulltos or cable rows to your chest. To thicken the middle part of your lats, you can do bent-over parallel barbell rows, dumbbell rows, or bar rows. An added advantage to doing dumbbell rows and cable rows is that they also build the posterior head of your deltoids, which is usually neglected.

The lower back is usually the most neglected area of the body, but it needs to be strong to prevent injuries from heavy lifting. If the lifter has a healthy back, I start him out with hyperextensions — first doing them on a flat bench, then later off a Roman chair. I also like doing good-morning exercises for the spinal erectors (lower-back muscles). After having done the basic exercises for six weeks to three months, dead lifts are recommended for the serious lifter. The dead lift works the legs and back in conjunction and is one of the three basic power lifts (the other two are the bench press and squat). The dead lift also coordinates all the back muscles in one lift and improves your grip, forearm, and traps. I have included stiff-legged deadlifts in the back section for simplicity's sake, but they really bomb the hams. I do not recommend single heavy cleans because they take so much skill and when they are not performed correctly, they can result in injury. However, light cleans in higher repetition strengthen the whole back and can help explosiveness.

There are many other back muscles, the rhomboid, infraspinatus, and teres major and teres minor, but for your purposes you need not worry about them. They will be worked by most of your rowing or chinning exercises.

47

The trapezoids (traps) are at the top of your back and connect to your shoulders. Shrugs and upright rows build them up. They are important in preventing shoulder and neck injuries.

Your back is one of the three crucial areas of your body in football. It is subjected to a pounding and needs to be built up to prevent injuries. It also needs to be strong for your blocking and tackling (these are grappling muscles); for real power you need a strong back. Strong lats also help the quarterback throw.

In basketball, your back takes a constant pounding from the hard court. You need to build up your lower back to prevent injuries; strengthening your back will help to give you power under the boards.

Baseball catchers have numerous back problems due to their stance. These problems can partially be prevented by building up your lower back. All players but, especially pitchers and catchers, need strong lats to help in throwing.

Soccer players' backs also take a pounding which can be helped by preventive weight-training exercises. Goalies could especially use lots of back work.

Swimmers' balance and power come principally from the back, and some strokes — especially the butterfly — utilize mainly the back muscles.

Wrestlers can both prevent back injuries and improve their power and explosiveness by building up their backs. Developing the lower back will help defend against the cradle, standups, and cross-body rides. With great lat strength, you will be able to squeeze the breath out of your opponent. They are tackling and grappling muscles.

Bodybuilders need a wide back for both the lat spread and general appearance. But this must not neglect their lower back both for their health and looks. They have to be very serious about developing all parts of their backs so they need to do a variety of back exercises.

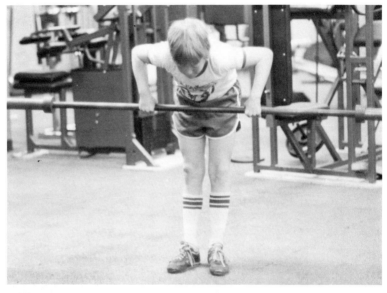

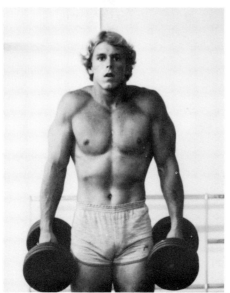

A1: Bent-Over Parallel Row
Hold the bar with a wide grip while you bend over, parallel to the ground. Pull the bar upwards until it strikes you in the chest, and then lower the bar slowly. This will develop the latissimus dorsi, which are important tackling muscles.

B1: Trapezoid Shrug
Grasp the dumbbells with your palms facing inward. Let your shoulders fall down, and then raise the shoulders without moving your arms.

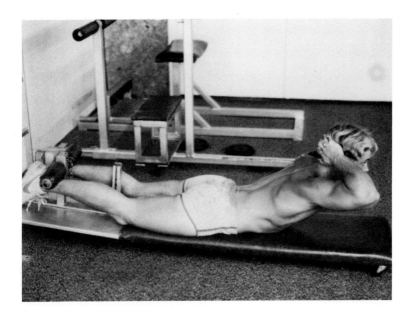

C1: Back Hyperextension

This exercise will require a
partner. Keep your hands
behind your head as your
partner holds your calves down.
Surge backwards, arching your
back to hyperextend yourself.
This will strengthen the lower
back and should be done in 3
sets of 20 to 25 repetitions.

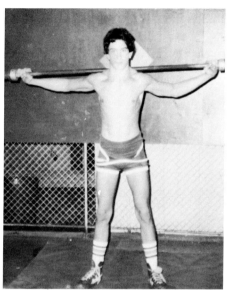 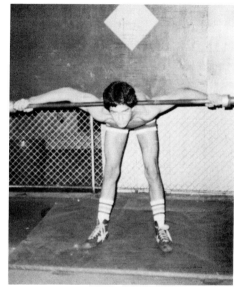

D1-2: Good Morning Exercise

Start with an empty bar when you begin your training program and then gradually build up the amount of weight you use. Place the bar behind your back from a standing position and then bend over until your back is parallel to the floor. Be sure that you are using a light amount of weight to avoid back strain. Build your routine up to 2 to 3 sets of 10 to 15 repetitions.

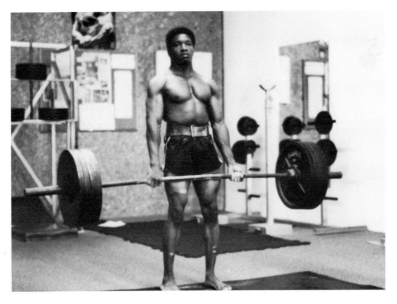

E1: Dead Lift

After you have performed the good morning exercise for a few weeks, move on to the dead-lift exercise. Address the bar with a grip slightly wider than your leg spread. Hold the bar with one palm facing frontwards and one facing backwards. Bend over and lift the bar to your waist, while keeping your arms straight. As you get the bar to this position, thrust your shoulders back and your chest out. This should be performed with light weight for the first few weeks, until the spinal erectors are strengthened. First try 15 repetitions. Then as your development progresses, you can decrease the repetitions and increase the amount of weight.

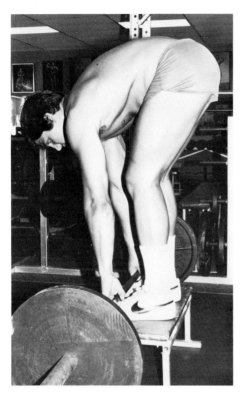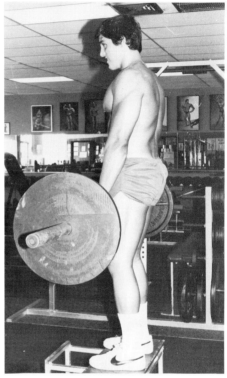

F1-2: Stiff-Legged Dead Lift
His best to stand on an elevated
platform with your legs almost
completely stiff. Bend down till
the barbells go below the
platform. Your back should be at
least parallel, if not lower; then
stand straight up. Make sure you
have really warmed up your back
and legs first. Avoid this exercise
if you have a back problem.

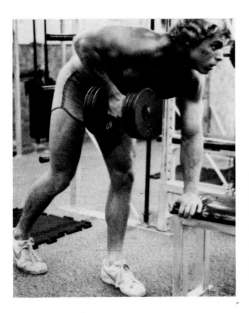

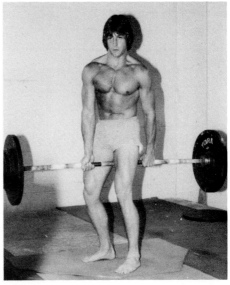

G1: One-Arm Dumbbell Row

Dumbbell rows help increase latissimus strength that is useful in tackling and also aid in flexibility due to the fuller range of motion that dumbbells provide. Keep both legs stiff and one arm placed on a bench or chair. Extend the dumbbell fully downward and then lift it back up until it hits your chest. Remember to keep the legs stiff and avoid cheating by bending your knees. This exercise should be repeated 12 times in sets of 3.

H1: Straddle

Straddle the barbell as you squat down to grip the bar with one palm up and one palm down. Then just stand up, being careful to keep your back straight as you bring the bar to your crotch. Then return to the starting position and repeat.

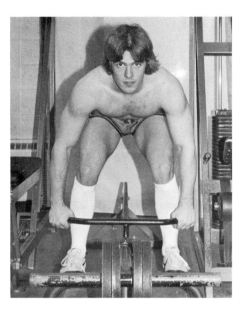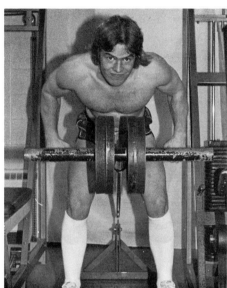

I1: T-Bar Row

Upward T-bar rows give the lats more power. Hold your hands on the bar and let the bar drop as you keep your back and knees slightly bent. Pull the bar up to your chest — being mindful of the full range of motion — letting the bar all the way down slowly and then pulling it to your chest. The form and the motion are more important than the amount of weight. Be careful not to use too heavy a weight at first. Also, avoid using your back — just the pulling motion.

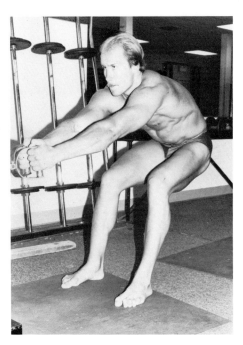 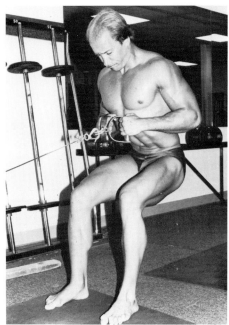

J1-2: Cable Row

Stand in a stooped position with a cable in each hand. At a few paces away from the plates, extend your arms fully out and pull them to your chest. Return to the starting position. You may also do this seated. This exercise will work your lats and the posterior head of your deltoids.

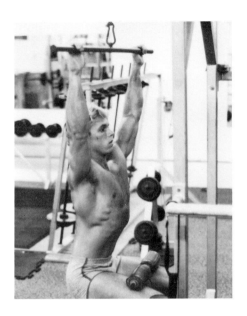 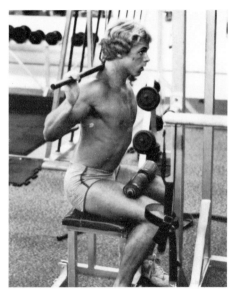

K1-2: Lat Pulldown

To start this exercise, kneel down with your hands holding the lat bar at the widest points. Pull down the bar behind your neck and allow the bar to return slowly to the outstretched position. Repeat. This is a great exercise for widening the lats. This exercise may be done also by pulling the bar down in front of you for variety.

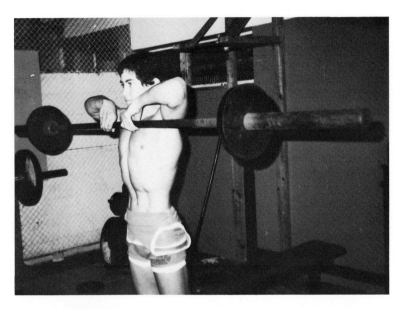

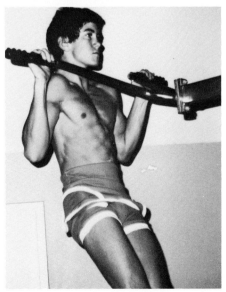

L1: Upright Row

Grasp the barbell with a narrow grip and raise the bar to a position even with your shoulders. Hold the bar in this position for a second or two while keeping your elbows pointed outward.

M1: Regular Chin-Up *(left)*

Grasp the bar with a palms-down position, shoulder width. Do not bounce or jerk your body going up.

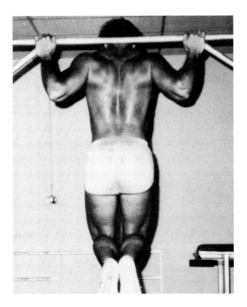

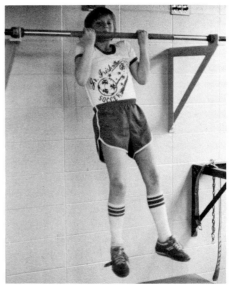

N1: Back-Grip Chin-Up *(above)*
This type of chin-up will develop
your lats, deltoids, and general
back area. Use a wide grip and
raise yourself until the back of
your head touches the bar.

O1: Underhand Chin-Up
Grasp the bar with a palms-up
hold, shoulder width.

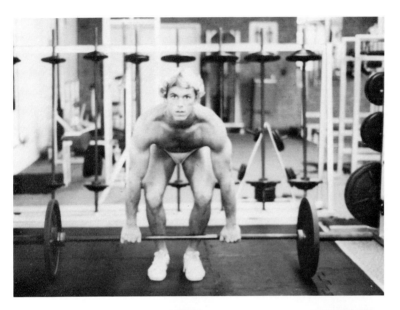

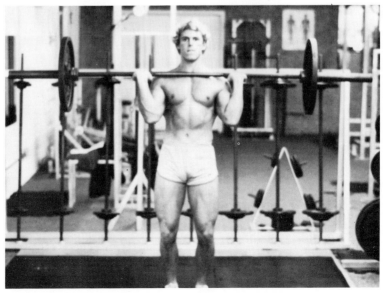

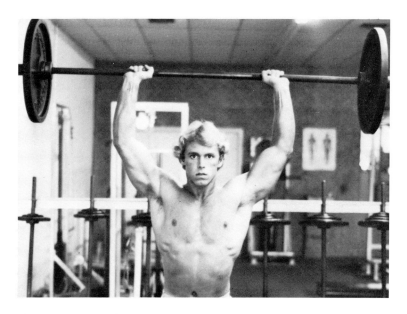

P1-3: Power Clean and Military Press

With your legs spread to shoulder width, grasp the bar so that your palms face the floor. Your thighs should be almost parallel to the floor as you explode into the next position illustrated. With your elbows pointing straight in front of you, spring off the floor onto the balls of your feet as you press the bar over your head. The press also works your deltoids and triceps.

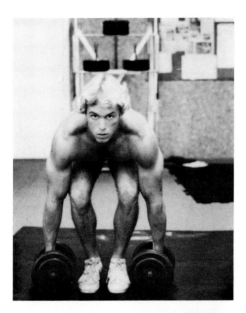
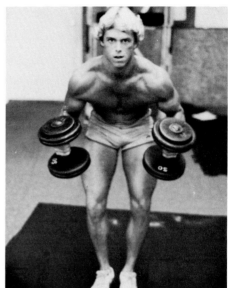
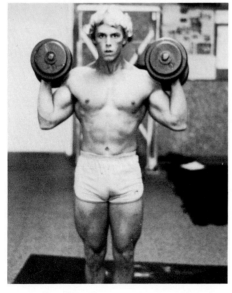
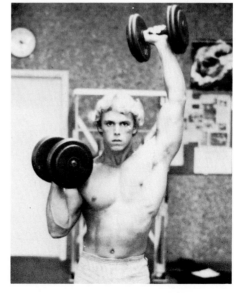

Q1-4: Dumbbell Clean and Press
The dumbbell clean and press improves power, explosiveness, strengthens the lower back, and builds all heads of the deltoids, plus the triceps, trapezoids, and wrists. Start by crouching in an almost seated position. Begin to clean the dumbbells by raising them over your shoulders. As soon as the dumbbells reach the top of your ankles, spring onto the balls of your feet to complete the motion. Next, press the dumbbells either simultaneously or by alternating arms.

R1-2: Clean and Jerk *(below)*
Start with the hands spread about shoulder width while keeping your back straight and your legs bent comfortably. Use the full power of your arms and shoulders as you clean the barbell on a vertical line to shoulder height. Balance the barbell on a line with your shoulders to prepare for the actual "jerk." Thrust the barbell upward from the shoulder position while scissoring your legs.

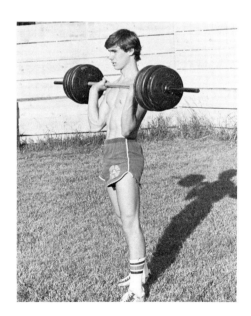
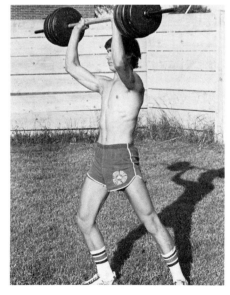

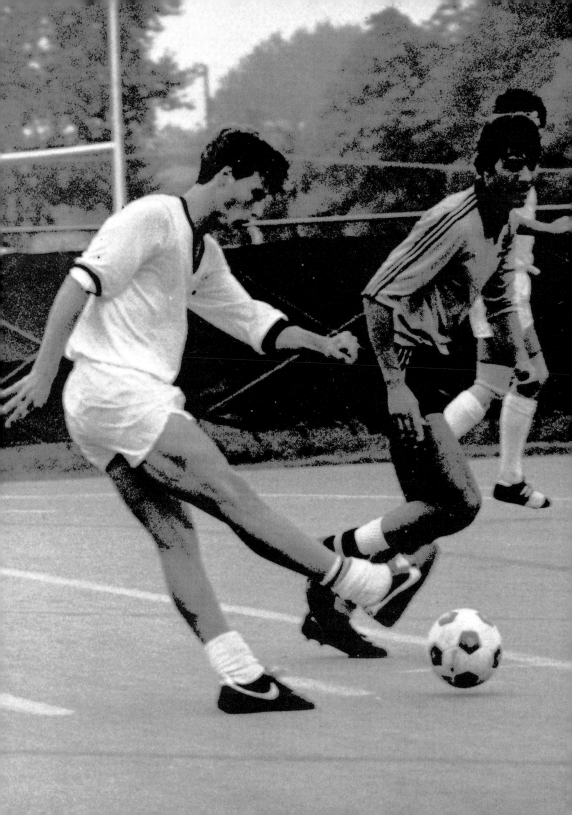

LEGS

Your legs are comprised of the gluteus maximus (hips); posterior thigh muscles (hamstring, on thigh biceps); anterior thigh muscles, which are generally called the quadriceps; and the calf, which is comprised of the gastrocnemius (major part of the calf and should be diamond shaped) and the soleus, which is the lower part of the calf. This is a simplification, since there are many more small muscle groups in your legs.

RUNNING IS NOT ENOUGH FOR YOUR LEGS! Running is great for cardiovascular conditioning, general body tone, and burning up calories. It is absolutely necessary for athletes, but it is not enough. You cannot support a big body on little pins. You need that weight training to build larger muscles. The main purpose for doing leg work is to prevent injuries. Eighty percent of the support for your knees comes from your quadriceps and hamstrings. You build those up significantly and reduce the chance of a serious injury like a torn ligament or cartilage by over 80 percent.

The secondary importance of leg work is speed. You are born with so much speed — you have it or you do not. However, you can improve your speed somewhat by building up your leg muscles.

The third importance of leg work is that exercises like squats will increase your whole body's strength, power, and cardiovascular condition.

The best exercise to develop leg size and strength is the squat. It not only works the glutes, quads, and hams, but it helps to expand the rib cage and get the blood flowing so as to help your whole body to glow. If there were only one exercise that I could do, it would be the squat. It works the legs and back in unison, as you do in sports. It is amazing how squats will build your appetite. High-repetition squats are also great for cardiovascular conditioning.

Variations of the basic parallel squat contained herein are the front squat (*dangerous*) and back squat. Next to the squat, the best overall exercise for your legs is the leg press. Squats and leg presses are better because they are natural pressing movements and work many parts of your legs together.

Leg extensions and curls are good for therapy, coming off an injury, a warm-up before squats or leg presses, and bringing out cuts (definition) for bodybuilding.

Your calves are the hardest muscle group to build up, mainly because you are using them constantly in walking, climbing stairs, and getting up from a seated position. Because they are so hard to build up, you really have to work through the pain. I recommend doing ten burning reps (you only start counting when you start to burn.)

Next to the prevention of injuries for football as well as other sports the second most important reason for weight training exercises for your legs is to improve your speed. In football, it could mean the difference between making the reception, outdistancing the defender or staying up with the receiver if you are a defensive back. For linemen, it could mean having the speed to pull out and lead the sweep, or if you are a defensive lineman, being able to pursue the runner. In basketball, you need speed to make the fast break or being able to stay up with the break. In baseball, improving your 60-yard dash speed from 7 seconds to 6.9 can mean the difference between batting .260 and .290. Improving your speed in baseball could make the difference between making a difficult catch or not. Wrestlers need speed to avoid a takedown as well as to make a takedown or escape. Soccer is probably the most obvious sport next to track in which speed is so crucial. Soccer players are like horses, constantly running and trying to outdistance the others, trying to get out in front and kick the ball. In swimming, half the game is leg kick.

Leg strength and power go hand in hand and are crucial to all sports. In football power and explosion comes from your legs and back in unison just as is developed by the squat. Your gluteus maximus (butt) is about the largest and most powerful muscle group in your body and is developed by squats and partially by leg presses. A big muscular butt (not fat) is important for sports, especially football, because it gives you the power to drive that opposing lineman off the line and helps the back break a tackle and drive for that extra yard.

In baseball leg strength is important because it gives you power for your hitting. That strength is also important for pitchers and can mean the difference of more than 10 mph in ball speed. This will become very evident to you if you just watch a pitcher wind up at the mound and go through the motion of his pitching. Especially watch how his thighs and hips are working.

Leg strength in basketball means the ability to jump for that rebound and to give you power to fight for that rebound. Al McGuire, former Marquette basketball coach and presently a TV commentator, has said he always wants his basketball players to have big muscular butts because it gives them an edge in their rebounding, both in power and in additional space between them and their opponents.

Soccer players need not only to be fast but have strength for kicking. There is no question but that a stronger leg will enable you to kick the ball harder and farther. Performing squats and leg presses will give you the stamina you need to keep on running and kicking. You will notice that I have also included lunges for soccer players because they will help your reverse speed.

Swimmers need incredibly strong quads and hams, and squats are the principal means to employ. Squats will help your stamina as well as strength.

Most bodybuilders and general fitness buffs always start their training with too much concentration on upper-body work and neglect their legs. As I have said earlier, you need to work all body parts so that your body is symmetrical.

Wrestlers need that leg strength and power for most of their moves. That leg strength is needed in stand-up switches, for deep penetration on takedowns, cross-body rides, and in defense against the cradle. The legs are also used in escapes and in control.

I have repeatedly warned that running is not enough. Running will help to give you general tone, burn up calories, and get your heart in shape, but it is not enough (unless you are an Olympic-class sprinter; now even they are doing squats and leg presses) to develop really good legs. Start working on those super legs before your upper body gets too big a head start, and you have to wear sweat pants on the beach!

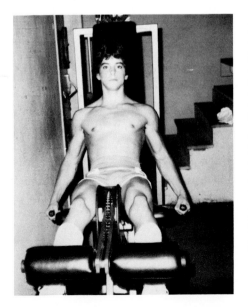

A1: Leg Extension (Nautilus)
In a seated position, place your feet behind the roller pads with your knees snug against the seat. Make sure to keep your head and your shoulders against the seat back. Straighten both of your legs smoothly. Pause. Slowly lower your resistance and repeat. It is important that you avoid tightly gripping the handles and gritting the teeth, tensing the neck or face muscles when you move.

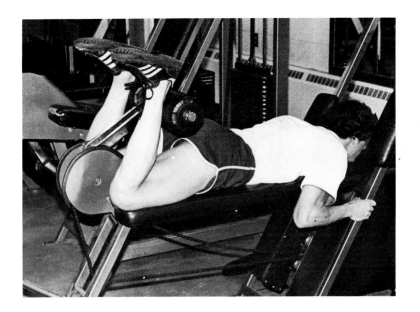

B1: Leg Curl (Nautilus)
Lie face down on the machine
and place your feet under the
roller pads with your knees just
over the edge of the bench.
Lightly grasp the handles to keep
your body from moving and then
curl your legs, trying to touch
your heels to your buttocks.
When your lower legs are
perpendicular to the bench, lift
your buttocks to increase your
movement. Then pause at the
point of full muscular
contraction. Slowly lower your
resistance and repeat the exercise.

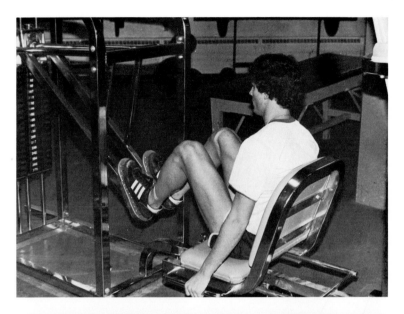

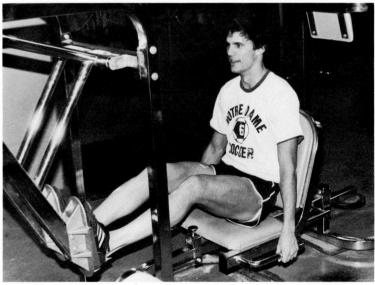

C1-2: Leg Press (Paramount)
Adjust the support chair until
your legs bend as indicated. Take
a deep breath and push with
your legs (uni- or bi-) until fully
extended, not locked. Exhale.
Return to the starting position.

D1-2: Leg Press
This old-fashioned leg-press
machine isn't recommended for
anyone recuperating from a knee
injury. Once again, fully extend
the leg 12 times a set, completing
3 sets. This machine does put
pressure on the knee, but can be
used in conjunction with other
leg exercises.

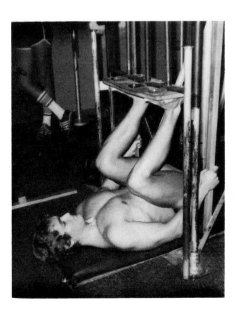
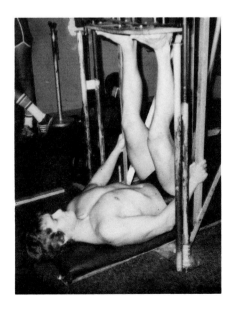

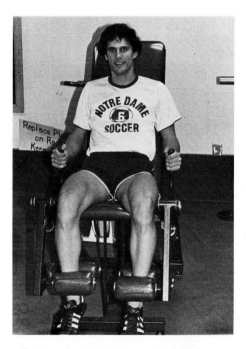

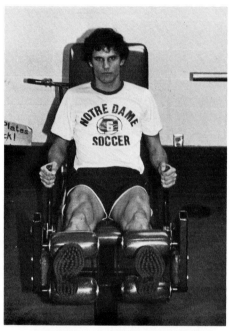

E1-2: Double-Knee Machine (Hydra-Gym Unilateral)
Fully extend your legs as hard and as fast as you can, then pull your legs back as hard and as fast as you can. This works both your quads and hams. Do as many reps as you can in a 20-second period.

F1-2: Regular Squat *(right)*
Place the weight behind the neck. This squat works the posterior and anterior thigh muscles, the gluteus maximus, and even the rib cage. Lower yourself slowly to avoid back injury, and don't bounce to keep unnecessary pressure off the knee.

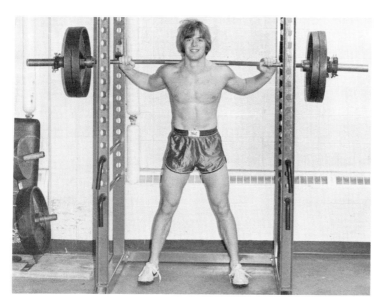

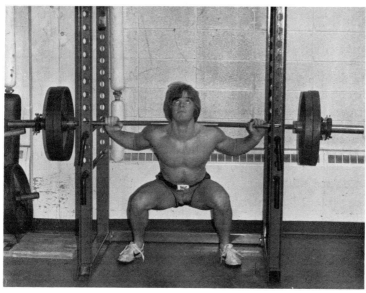

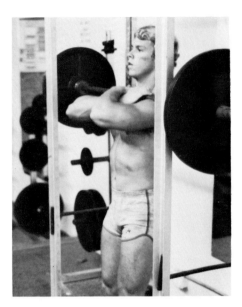 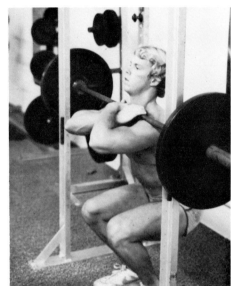

G1-2: Front Squat

Front squats will help you
strengthen your quadriceps.
Start by resting the weight on
your shoulders in an upright
position, arms are crossed to
hold the barbell as prepare to
squat. Lower yourself until your
thighs are parallel to the floor.
Remember to keep your back
straight and your head up while
you lower yourself to the down
position. Don't bounce into the
lower position. The success of
this exercise relies on lowering
yourself slowly.

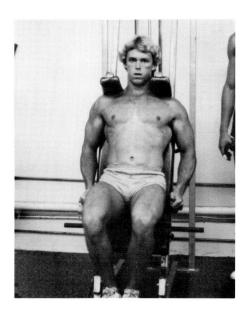
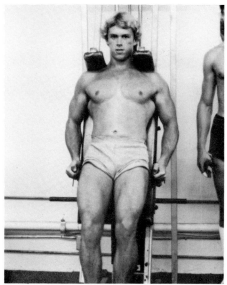

H1-2: Hack Squat

Grip the bar behind your back in a downward position and then raise up to a three-quarters position. Then move down until your thighs are parallel to the ground. Make sure you only come three-quarters of the way up. This exercise pumps the quadriceps (anterior thigh muscles) as well as some posterior thigh muscles effectively. Some bodybuilders prefer this exercise to the regular squat because it does not work your glutes.

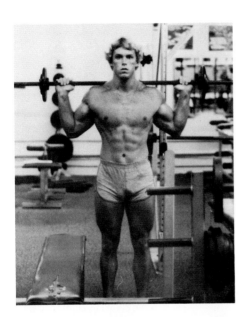

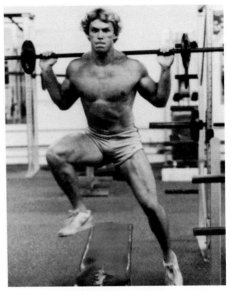

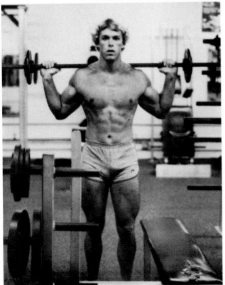

I1-3: Side Jump

Rest the bar on your back and, while raising your legs one at a time, jump sideways over a bench. Then reverse the jump. You should do this in sets of twenty. Make sure you start with a light weight and low bench. This exercise will work your abductors, adductors, and help your lateral speed. This exercise is especially good for baseball infielders.

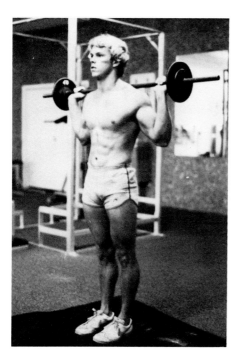 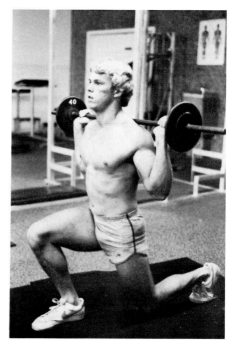

J1-2: Bar Lunge

Stand straight up with the bar resting on your back. Extend one leg forward and bend down until the opposite leg is almost touching the ground. Then stand up straight and lunge forward with the other leg. This exercise effectively pumps your thighs, especially the glute-ham tie-in.

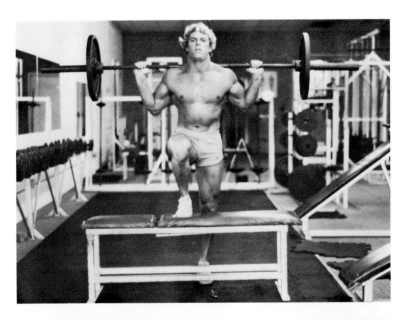

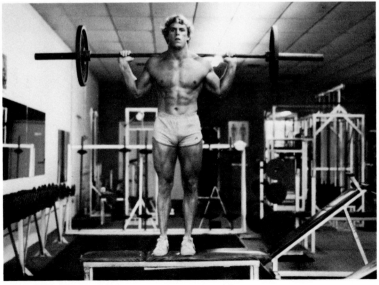

K1-2: Step-Up

This is as easy as walking up and down the stairs. With weight in position as pictured, just step up and down on a step.

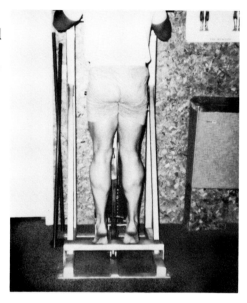

L1: Toe Raise

The calves are the target of this exercise performed using this toe-raise machine. The development of the calves can increase a player's speed and quickness, and toe raises work on the calves with quick results. Try for a full extension as you thrust upward onto your toes. Do this exercise in sets of 20.

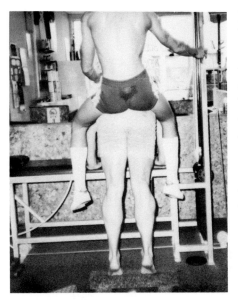

M1: Donkey Toe Raise

Donkey toe raises are a more difficult exercise because of the weight's closer proximity to the calves. Have a partner sit on your back as you brace yourself over a table. Thrust upward onto your toes a minimum of 20 repetitions a set. You should feel that good "burning sensation" in the calves at least 10 times to utilize this exercise effectively.

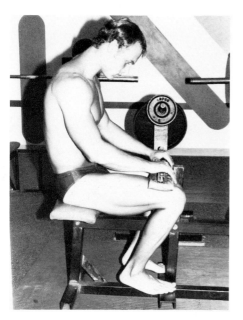 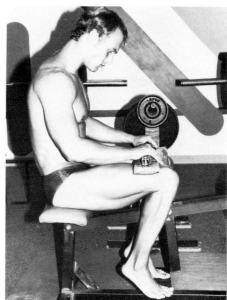

N1-2: Seated Calf-Toe Raise

Wedge your knees under the
padded bar and move your heels
up and down as far as possible.
This exercise works your soleus,
or the lower part of your calves.
Make sure you do at least ten (10)
burning repetitions.

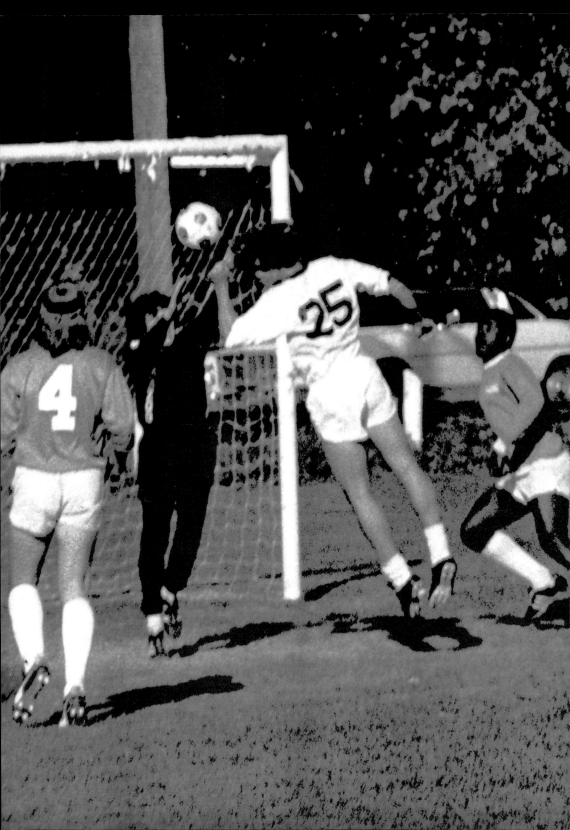

NECK

The neck is the most susceptible part of the body to injury. It just wasn't built to take the abuse it gets in football. It is taking tremendous pressure in blocking and tackling even though the old spearing is illegal. You continually hear coaches yell "stick your face in his chest," and you better believe that your neck is taking the brunt of the pressure. But it's not just linemen and linebackers whose necks are being pressured. Wide receivers and running backs probably receive the most neck injuries. A very sad but notable example of this is Daryl Stingley of the New England Patriots who was a wide receiver a few years ago. A dangerous and unfortunate tackle to his neck caused paralysis, and he will probably never walk again! It is crucial for football players to build up their neck muscles. The two machines I like the best are the Hyrda-Gym and Nautilus machines. If you don't have these, there are many exercises in this chapter that you can substitute for.

Baseball and basketball players and swimmers don't usually sustain neck injuries, so for them the indirect work the neck gets from military presses and upright rows is enough. This isn't to say they should avoid all neck work.

Soccer players don't normally sustain injuries to their necks, but an ounce of prevention is worth a pound of cure. Thirty seconds, two or three times a week on the neck machine can mean a lot to your heading game.

You almost always see wrestlers with huge necks, for they are constantly using them in wrestling and have long known the importance of building them up to prevent injuries and to help them wrestle better.

Besides the importance of building up your neck to prevent injuries, those muscles are used in bridging, stabilization against the nelson, and ducking under a takedown.

Generally you don't see bodybuilders working their necks because too big a neck is not an attractive body part, and your neck is about the easiest part to build up. When you do any trap work like shrugs or upright rows, you are building up your neck indirectly. Your neck also gets stimulation from any form of military presses.

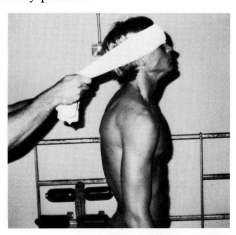

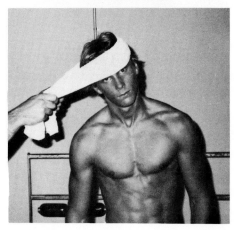

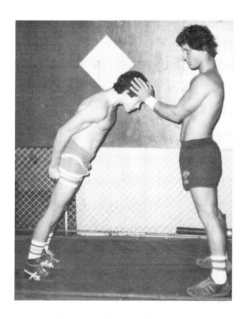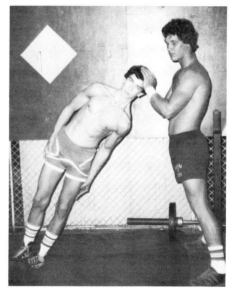

A1-2: Towel Neck Exercise
First start by having your partner place the towel behind the back of your neck and apply pressure toward the front. Try to touch the back of your head to your back while the tension is being applied. Now try the same exercise with the towel on the back of the head and at each side. Attempt to move your head in the opposite direction of the tension, bringing your head forward to your chest or your ear to your shoulder.

B1-2: Isometric Neck Exercise
This exercise is designed to put constant pressure on the neck muscles while the exerciser is leaning into the arms of his partner. The neck muscles are doing the work supporting the person's weight. Just stand stiff and lean into your partner's hands while letting all of your weight be supported by the neck muscles. This exercise should be done in directions to the right, left, and straight ahead.

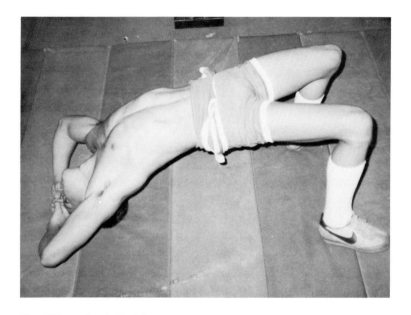

C1: Wrestler's Bridge

Place your feet flat and firm as you bridge yourself so that your feet and head are the only parts of your body in contact with the floor. When you reach this position, roll back, forth, and sideways to get the most out of the exercise.

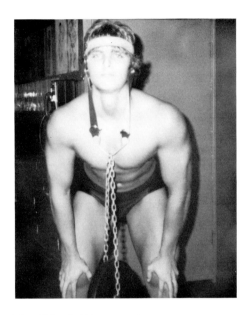

D1: Neck Harness
Bend your back as you stand in a
crouched position. Lower your
head and then raise it while just
utilizing your neck muscles. Be
careful not to use too much
weight in this exercise.

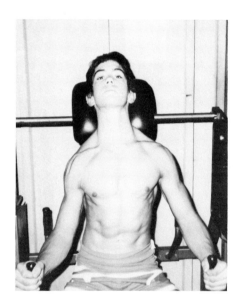 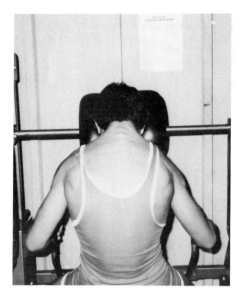

E1-4: Neck Machine (Nautilus 4-Way)
(posterior extension)
Adjust the seat so your Adam's apple is in line with the axis of the cam. The back of your head should contact the middle of the pads. Stabilize your torso by lightly grasping the handles. Extend your head as far back as possible and pause. Slowly return to the stretched position and repeat.

(anterior flexion)
Face the machine and adjust the seat so your nose is in the center of the pads. Stabilize your torso by lightly gripping the handles. Smoothly move your head toward your chest. Pause. Then slowly return to the stretched position and repeat.

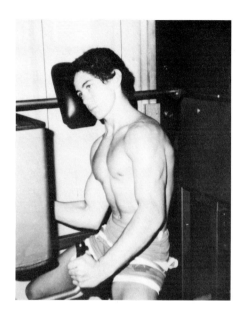 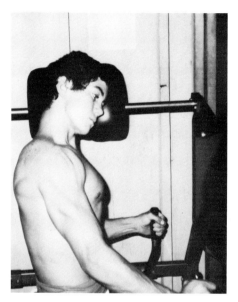

(lateral contraction)

Your left ear should be in the center of the pads. Stabilize your torso by lightly grasping the handles. Smoothly move your head toward your left shoulder. Pause. Keep your shoulders square and then slowly return to the stretched position and repeat. Reverse the procedure for the right side.

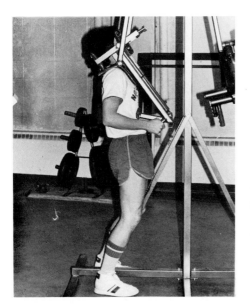
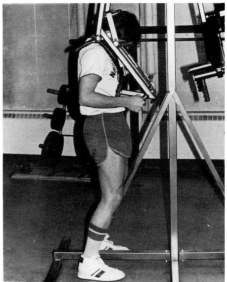
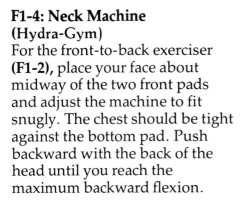

F1-4: Neck Machine
(Hydra-Gym)
For the front-to-back exerciser **(F1-2)**, place your face about midway of the two front pads and adjust the machine to fit snugly. The chest should be tight against the bottom pad. Push backward with the back of the head until you reach the maximum backward flexion.

Then **push** directly forward into the pads until you reach the maximum forward flexion. For the side-to-side exerciser **(F3-4)**, place the head about midway between the two sets of pads (you should be able to see just over the bar that holds the cylinders) and adjust the head

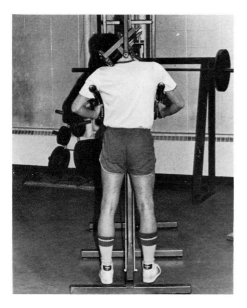 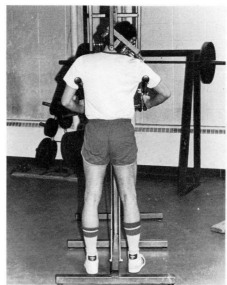

pads to fit snugly against the
sides of the head. The arms
should be over the two round
bars, and you should grip the
two grippers at the end of the
round bars. Pull the head from
side to side, getting the
maximum range while
maintaining the body as rigidly
as possible.

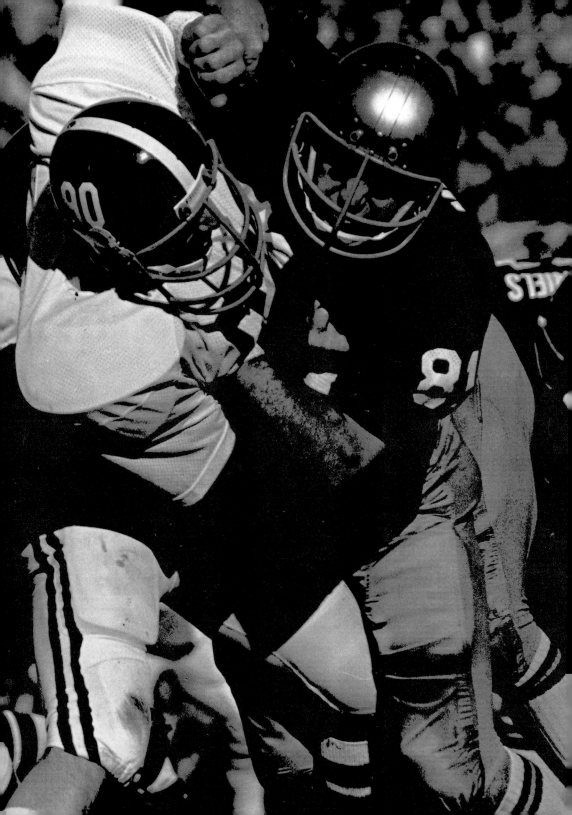

ARMS & WRISTS

Although the biceps are one of the least important muscles for football players, when we have plenty of time in the off-season we can spare a little time to build them up. You might be able to put on a couple of pounds of muscle there. The biceps only comprise 40 percent of the upper arm, while the triceps account for the other 60 percent.

The triceps are more important for football because they are used in blocking, especially pass blocking, in pushing off a blocker, and, of course, in stiff arming. The quarterback uses his triceps in his throwing. That's why I include lots of tricep work like dips in his routines. The forearms and wrists are more important than biceps for footballers because they are used more in grabbing a back, tossing aside a blocker, throwing a forearm shiver, and even for the receivers who need strong wrists to make difficult receptions.

Basketball players need strong wrists both to hold onto the ball and to help them steal the ball. Strong wrists and forearms also help in their shot. For basketball players the bicep isn't crucial, but in the off-season should be built up as part of a total body workout, and it will help in holding onto the ball. The triceps are used in shooting, but during the season the work they get from military presses is sufficient.

Baseball players, especially pitchers, should be concerned with building up arms to prevent elbow problems (tendonitis and hyperextension of the elbow). Building up the biceps, triceps, and forearms reduces the chance of a disabling elbow problem from occurring. Building up the forearms and triceps will help you grip the bat and hit better. Strengthening the arms will also help pitchers throw harder and with more control.

The arms are not too important for soccer players, except maybe the goalie. Therefore, we only directly work them in the off-season when we have plenty of time to do total body workouts. Arm strength is secondary for swimmers too, so only minimal work is included here.

Wrestlers should also be concerned with building up their arms to prevent torn biceps and hyperextended elbows. Arm strength is used generally in takedowns, reversals, and in control for gripping. Specifically, you use the triceps in breaking wrist tie-ups, arm extensions, wrist rides, and cradles. You also use your arms in recovering to all fours from the takedown. The forearms are used in wrist and ankle control and in arm tie-ups.

For those of you interested in bodybuilding, your arms are likely your biggest concern. Big arms make a man look strong and macho. The maximum you can develop your arms is based on heredity and bone structure, as I discussed earlier. The maximum you can "naturally" develop your arms is 10 to 11 inches larger than your wrist. Remember that your triceps are the largest part of your upper arm, so don't just do curls and expect to have huge arms. Your triceps have three heads: (1) inner (medial) head, (2) outer (long), head, and (3) side (lateral) head. All three of these heads should be worked to get your maximum arm size. I like the close-grip bench press for complete development of your triceps. A word of caution in tricep work; many people have sustained elbow problems in doing their tricep work, especially in extensions, so it is important to do lots of warm-ups and do your specific tricep work after your presses.

When it comes to biceps, my favorite exercise is the dumbbell incline curl. With this, you get both a full development of your bicep as well as peaking it. The stretch you get from doing the curl on an incline board is invaluable. I like the dumbbells because they allow more range of motion and develop the arms and secondarily work the forearms equally.

Beginners should not include specific forearm work because the indirect work they get from curls is sufficient at this stage of their development. For more advanced trainees, I prescribe both wrist curls and reverse curls for their forearms. The forearms consist of a number of cable-like muscles that have the function of pronators, which rotate the head inward, and supinators, which rotate it outward. There are a number of smaller and less prominent muscles in your arms, like the brachialis but we need not go into them. But don't worry. The brachialis and others are being worked by your dumbbell curls.

A last word of warning in training your arms — avoid preacher curls. They are a good bodybuilding exercises for biceps but can be very harmful to the elbows and can bring on tendonitis. If you are using 100 pounds on your preacher curls, you have 20,000 pounds of pressure per square inch on your elbows! An athlete, especially a pitcher or quarterback, can't afford that!

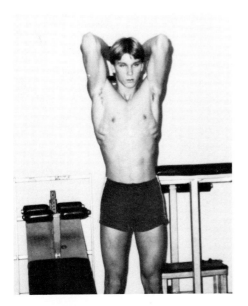 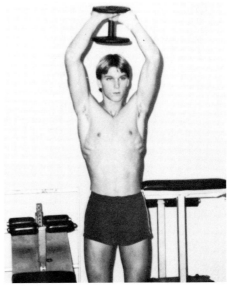

A1-2: Standing or Seated Tricep Extension

In this exercise, you can choose a standing or sitting position, whichever is more comfortable for you. Start by gripping the dumbbell with both hands. Lower it behind your head as low as it will go. After you have reached this low point, slowly press the dumbbell over your head, making sure that your elbows are pointed inward as you press upward.

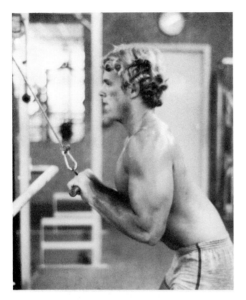 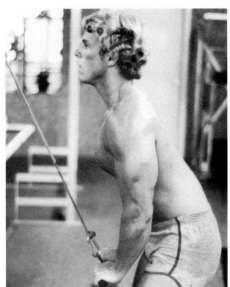

B1-2: Tricep Pushdown
Stand erect, narrow grip on bar, palms down or up, and elbows fixed at your sides. Take a deep breath and force the bar down until the arm is fully extended. Exhale. Return.

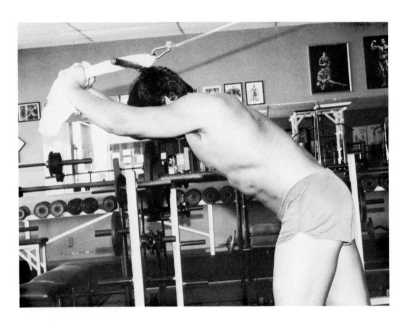

C1: Cable Tricep Pull

You can use either a towel or a small bent bar to perform this exercise. Take a few steps forward from the cable and extend your arms all the way back. Bring the towel at least two-thirds of the way forward, well past your head. This exercise effectively bombs your triceps.

D1-2: Lying Tricep Extension

In a prone position, grip the easy-curl bar with your hands close together. Hold the bar over your forehead and press it upwards to a position directly over your chest. Make sure you extend your arms completely.

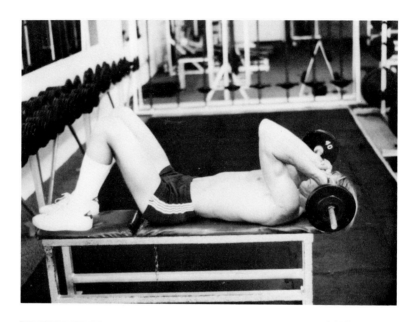

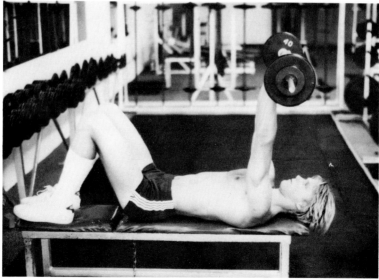

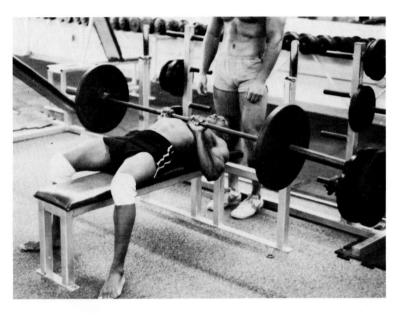

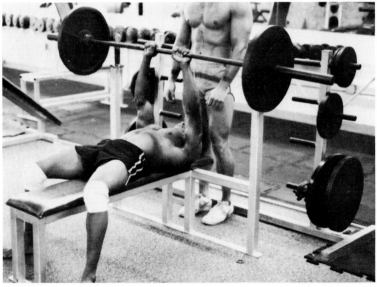

E1-2: Close-Grip Bench Press
(left)
Use a narrow grip, and lower the bar to your lower pectoral area. Keep your back in contact with the bench as you explode and press the bar into the air.

F1-2: One-Arm French Curl
Again you can choose the standing or sitting position. Grasp the dumbbell in a palms-up grip with the dumbbell horizontal to the floor. Lift it over your shoulder, twisting it so that it is now in a vertical position. Drop the dumbbell behind the shoulder, remembering to keep your arm and elbow pointed straight ahead. Complete the exercise by pressing the dumbbell straight over your shoulder.

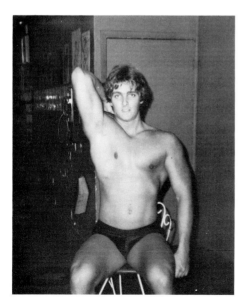
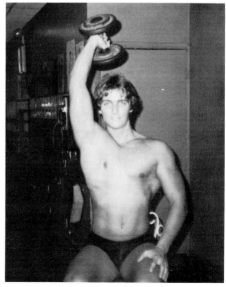

G1: Straight Dip
Remain straight on the parallel
bars, and lower yourself until
your shoulders and the bars are
almost even. Then press straight
up until you reach your starting
position again.

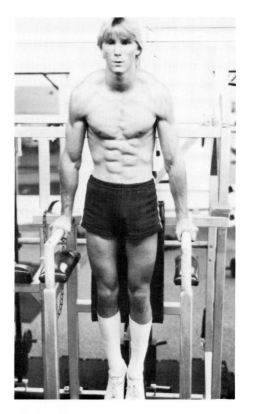

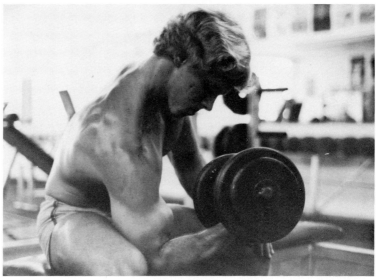

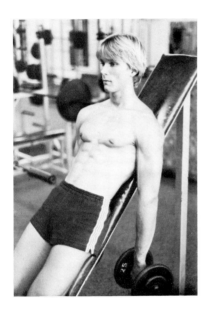

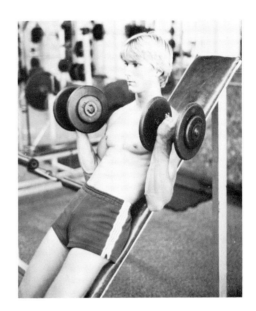

I1-2: Dumbbell Incline Curl

These curls may be done with both arms together or one at a time. Hold the dumbbells with a palms-up grip in a resting position, with your arms fully extended downward. Curl the dumbbells straight up until they almost touch your shoulders.

H1: One-Arm Concentrated Curl

(left)

Start with a palms-up grip; touch your upper arm to the same-side leg. Proceed to curl the dumbbell until you touch your shoulder.

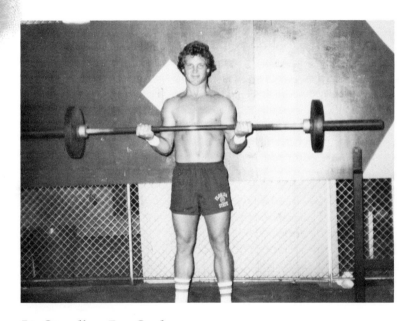

J1: Standing Bar Curl

Grip the straight bar in a wide or narrow grip while standing straight, and then curl the bar to your shoulders. If you are using a heavy weight, you can cheat by bending your back slightly. Be careful. This exercise puts strain on the lower back.

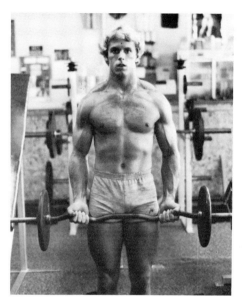 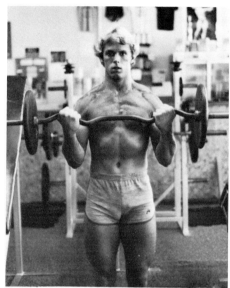

K1-2: Standing Cheating Curl (with easy-curl bar)

With back straight, stand stiffly and with arms held close in, simply curl straight up to your shoulders from the down position. You may cheat a little on the last repetition, but be careful, for you could hurt your back by doing so.

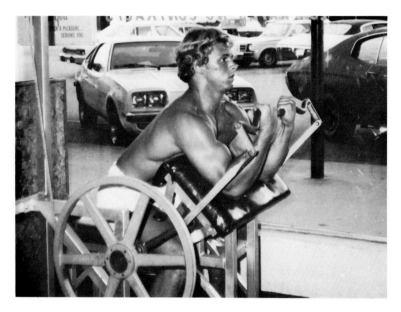

L1: Preacher Curl

Rest your elbows on the preacher bench with the arms fully extended. Curl up toward your shoulder. This will fill in the lower part of your bicep. It is also called the Scott curl after Larry Scott, who popularized it. Avoid if you have tendonitis.

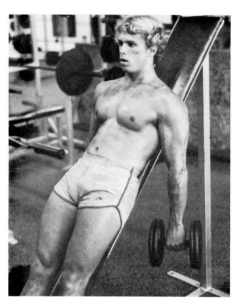 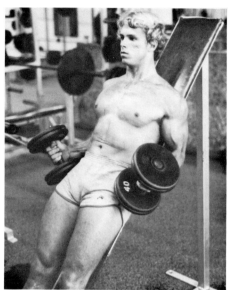

M1-2: Supinating Curl

In this exercise, you should be
lying on an incline bench with
your arms extended down, glued
to your sides. Curl the dumbbells
almost to your shoulders. Make
sure the bench is at a 45° angle
with your feet elevated. Notice
that you should supinate, or turn,
the dumbbells as you bring them
up toward your shoulder. This
turning up of the dumbbells
gives an extra peak to your
biceps. The stretch you get from
the incline dumbbells greatly
builds up your biceps.

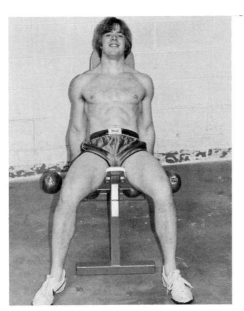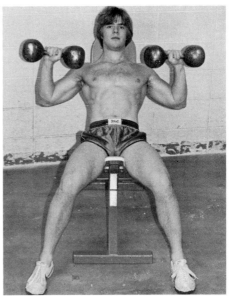

N1-2: Pronating Curl

Preferably from an incline bench, hold the dumbbells while at the fully stretched-down position with your palms facing up. As you curl the dumbbells up, turn them at your hip so that when you reach the top of the movement, your palms will be facing down and slightly out. This is both a peaking movement as well as being great for the forearms.

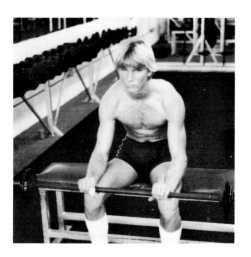

O1: Wrist Curl (down position)
These curls will strengthen the wrists and forearms, vulnerable areas for tight ends and wide receivers. Hold the bar or dumbbell in your hands with a palms-down grip. Relax your wrists so that they drop as far as they will go, then flex and raise your wrists as high as you can.

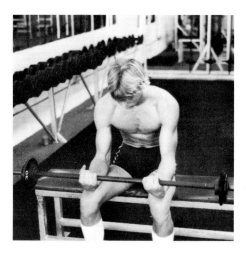

P1: Wrist Curl (up position)
This curl will help the wrists and forearms too, but it adds an extra twist to strengthen the hands and fingers. Rest your forearms on your thighs while holding the bar with your palms facing upward. Let the bar drop to the end of your fingers and then roll your fingers up, grabbing the bar in your palms again. Conclude the exercise by flexing your wrists as high as you can.

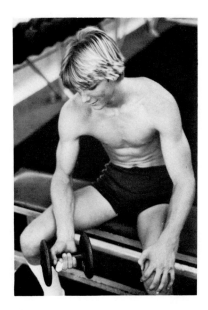 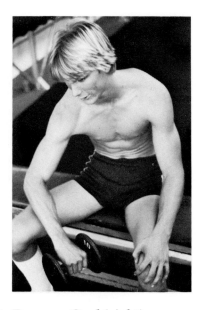

Q1-2: Wrist Curl, Flip Flop *(above)*
Hold a dumbbell with the palms up and the forearm resting on your leg. Flip the wrist so that the dumbbell and your palm are facing down. Repeat to the starting position and do sets of 15 reps.

R1-4: Reverse Curl *(right)*
Take your choice of using either an easy-curl bar or a dumbbell. Holding either with a narrow or wide palms-down grip, curl it to your shoulders. These curls are aimed at developing the forearms.

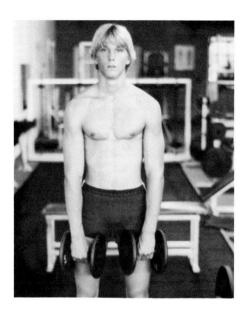
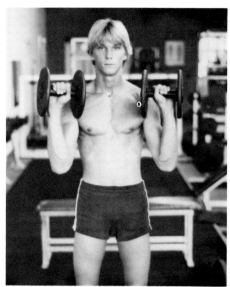

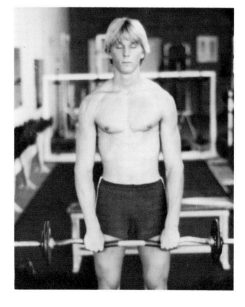
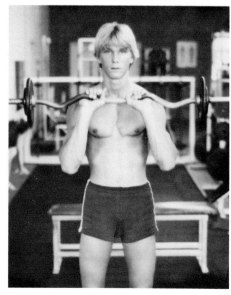

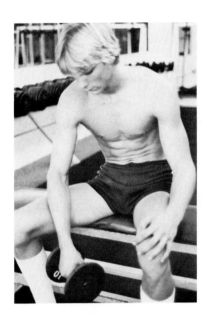 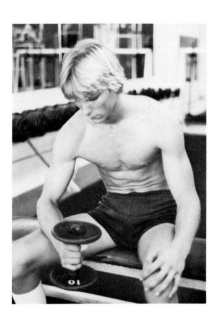

S1-2: Sideways Curl

With your arm resting on your
knee or a bench, holding the
dumbbell sideways, extend the
dumbbell fully up and down.

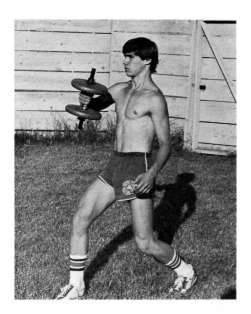

T1: Lunge Curl

This was popularized by Rubin
Carter of the Denver Broncos.
Tremendously helpful in
improving your pass rush.
Lunge forward on the right leg,
curling the right arm to the left
shoulder. Repeat with the left.
This builds power and explosion
in the lower back and thighs,
building up the forearms, wrists,
biceps, and anterior heads of the
deltoids.

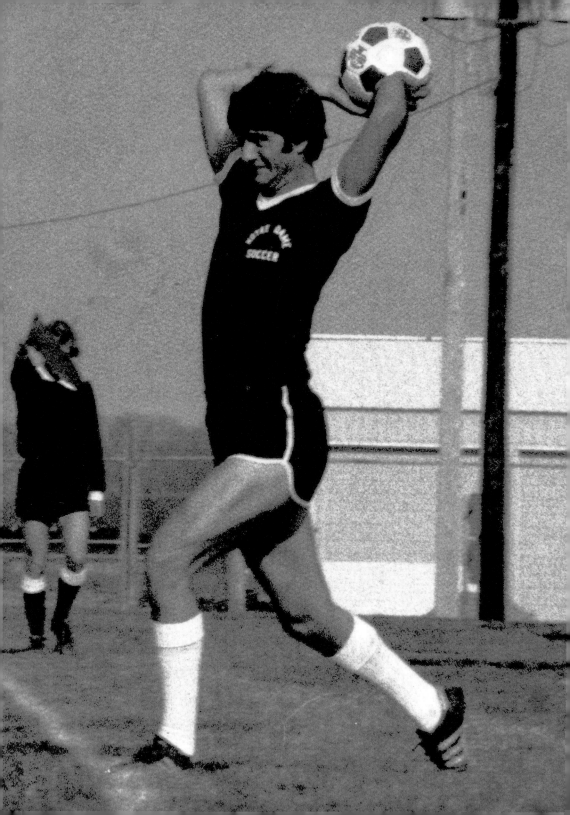

CHEST

The largest part of the chest consists of the pectorals, major and minor. The rib cage is also considered part of the chest. You are at a prime time in your life when you can make great gains in expanding your rib cage. After age 21, it will be extremely difficult to expand your rib cage. All heavy breathing exercises, such as squats and pullovers, will expand your rib cage.

The chest is not one of the prime areas of concern in football. You don't often hear of a ripped pec in football. However, the upper chest and pec-delt tie-in areas do take a lot of pounding in blocking and tackling. Building up that pec-delt tie-in area will give more stability to the shoulder and help prevent shoulder separations. I look at the chest as an area where I can pack muscle on a boy, which means weight — so important to linemen. A great advantage of doing heavy breathing exercises such as pullovers is that by expanding the rib cage you give your lungs more room to expand so you don't tire out so much in the fourth quarter.

You will note from my programs that I don't stress the regular bench press for football but prefer the dumbbell incline press. The incline press both more approximates the angle you come off the line and develops the more important muscle groups than the bench (you don't play football standing straight up). More importantly, the incline develops the upper pecs, which take more of a pounding than the major pecs, and the pec-delt tie-in area, which helps to stabilize the shoulders. I stress dumbbells more than barbells because you don't play football with a stick in your hand; you use your arms independently in football as you do with dumbbells. Also, dumbbells allow for more range of motion, more than any fancy machine, and that stretching increases flexibility. In addition, dumbbells develop the secondary muscle groups better, improve your grip, and strengthen your forearms.

When I get into more advanced training programs, I will use the close-grip bench as a supplement because it is a great developer of the triceps, which are used in blocking, especially pass blocking. I also use the close-grip bench for quarterbacks because their triceps are so important in their throwing.

Although I don't consider the bench press a great chest exercise (only 30 to 38 percent of the exercise works the major pec; the rest of it works the front head of your deltoids and your triceps), I have included it in this section because most people consider it a major chest exercise and because it is a compound exercise that among other things does work the pecs. The wider out you hold the bar, the more you work the pecs; the closer in you hold your hands, the more tricep work you get.

Baseball players shouldn't be overly concerned with their chests because it is not that important to their playing. I have included incline presses because the muscle groups they build up, upper pecs and pec-delt tie-in area, will help in hitting power. I sometimes use the bench press for baseball players as an overall upper-body power exercise. I do use close-grip bench presses for pitchers because that will help in their pitching.

Pectoral strength is also not very important to basketball players. However, it is an area in which we can pack muscle that will be helpful in rebounding. I use dumbbell incline flies in basketball because the areas built up by that exercise, the upper pecs and pec-delt tie-in, are important in defense. The range of motion in this exercise is great and will really help in giving you the strength to move your arms all over and in front of the man you are guarding. Pullovers also help in conditioning, so your lungs have more room to expand.

Soccer players also shouldn't be overly concerned with their chests. During the off-season, when we have plenty of time, we work on developing the chest as part of an overall lifting program but don't worry about it during the season. Building up the chest does have the benefit of giving you a cushion in collisions, and in trapping, and the pullovers, which expand that rib cage, will help to keep you from tiring out so fast.

Chest strength is extremely important for swimmers. All the basic strokes utilize the chest greatly, and expanding the rib cage is central in increasing wind and stamina for those grueling long races. I suggest crossover flies and pullovers as central exercises in and out of season.

In wrestling, the pectorals are used in recovering to all fours, in the breakdown, and in initiating standups. Pecs are used along with the delts, arms, and legs in defense (clearing cover) and in the overhook series and cradles. I also prefer dumbbell incline presses for wrestlers for independent development, greater stretch for flexibility, and improvement in grip and forearm power they afford.

For those of you interested in bodybuilding, the chest is probably the second most popular body part. Building a big chest will make a boy look like a man, and manliness and big chests have long been equated. I feel that the two best chest exercises are the dumbbell incline press coupled with either the decline press or forward dip. The incline press develops the upper chest and the decline and forward dip both work the lower and outer chest. I like an angle of about 38° for the incline. Once you get over 45°, you are getting too much deltoid. For more advance lifters I add either flat flies or incline flies to build up the outer chest and square off the pecs. But I wouldn't worry about that until you are a lot more advanced. Don't concentrate on just your chest. Your whole body needs to be developed equally. If you just concentrate on one body part, you will look very funny. Imagine a 17-year-old boy who has a 45-inch chest but only 19-inch thighs.

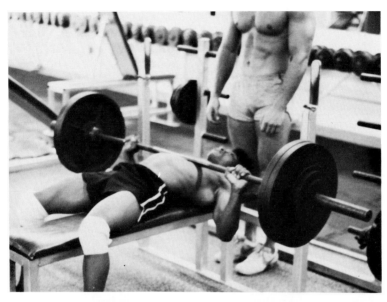

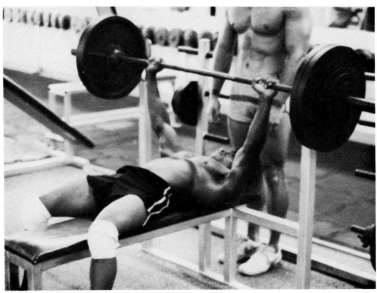

A1-2: Bench press *(left)*
Keep the hands at shoulder
length while performing the
same instructions for the
wide-grip press. This will
develop the deltoids, triceps, and
pectorals.

B1-2: Barbell Incline press
(below)
While at a 45° angle, press the
bar upwards with an exhaling
breath, pausing to lock your
arms in an extended position,
and then lower the bar back
down to the top of your
pectorals. The incline press is
also beneficial for building the
pectoral-deltoid tie-in — an area
of the upper chest that the bench
press does not develop.

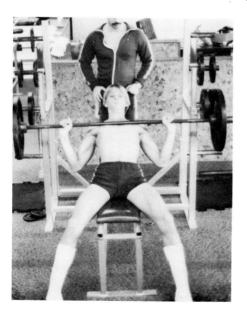
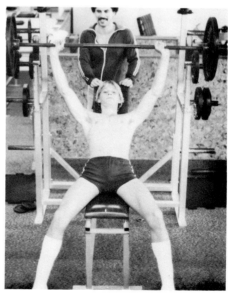

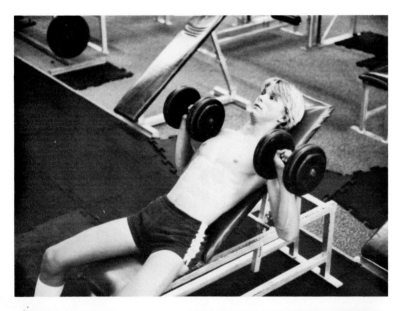

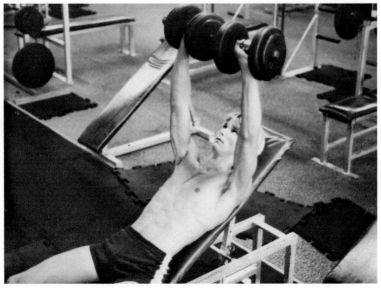

C1-2: Dumbbell Incline Press
(left)
The dumbbell incline press is designed to strengthen the upper pectorals and triceps. It is especially effective for the pectoral-deltoid tie-in. Starting with the dumbbells wide apart yet touching your shoulders, press the dumbbells upwards until they are closer than at the start.

D1: Dumbbell Decline Press
This exercise works the lower pectorals as well as the anterior head of the deltoids and triceps. You reverse your position from the incline, thereby having your head at the bottom and feet in the air. Hold the dumbbells wide at the base, touching your shoulders, and press them up, narrow at the top.

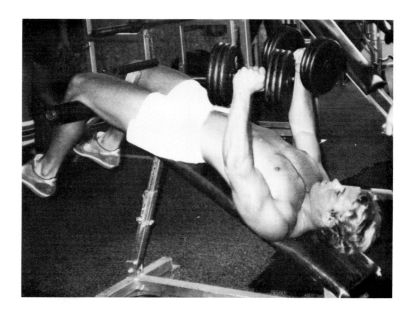

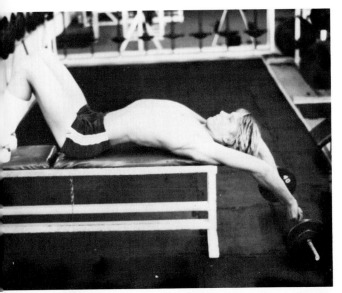

E1-4: Easy-Curl Pullover and Dumbbell Pullover

Lying either straight or across a bench with your head over the edge, pull the bar off the ground over your head to a position over the top of your pectorals, keeping the hip in contact with the bench and the bar or dumbbell from touching your pecs. Avoid using heavy weight for the pullover, for this will cause you to cheat by bending the elbows. Keep the rib cage relaxed, so you can stretch the entire rib structure.

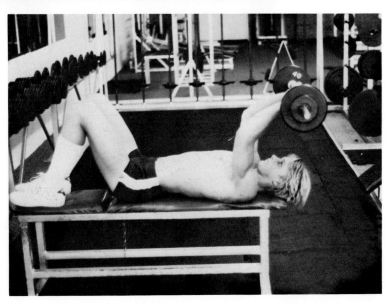

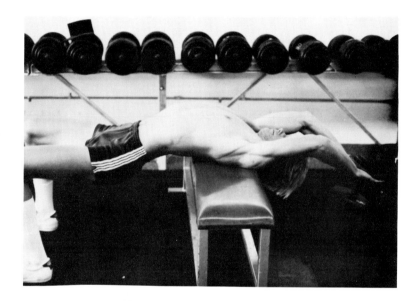

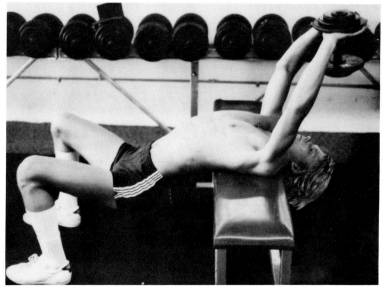

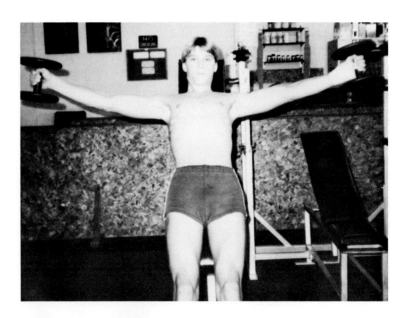

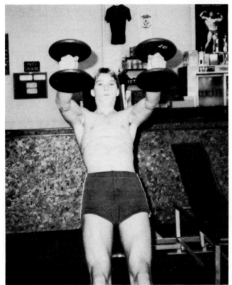

F1-2: Incline Fly
With your back resting on an incline of about 45°, extend your arms out as far as they will go, holding the dumbbells with a palms-up grip. Keeping your elbows slightly bent, bring the dumbbells two-thirds to three-quarters of the way across the chest. Don't lift the dumbbells all the way up and together, for that takes the tension off. This is great for developing the upper and outer pectorals.

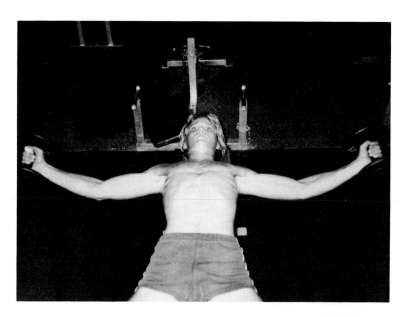

G1-2: Lying Flat Fly

While lying flat on the bench with a dumbbell in each hand, extend your arms below the bench with your elbows slightly bent. Bring the two dumbbells up toward your chest (two-thirds of the way). You do not want to bring the dumbbells together because it takes the tension off. This exercise works to square off your middle pectorals (the major part of your chest) and the front and side heads of your deltoids.

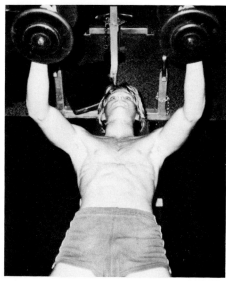

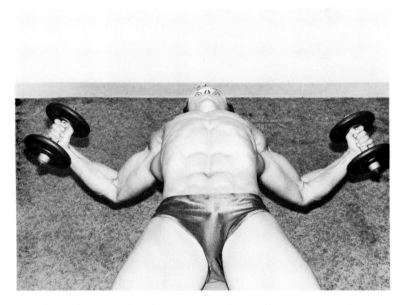

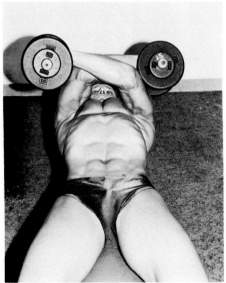

H1-2: Lying Crossover Fly
While lying on a flat bench,
extend your arms below the
bench with your elbows slightly
bent. Bring the dumbbells across
your chest so that they cross each
other. This is a more advanced
exercise than the regular flat fly.
It also works the inner pecs.

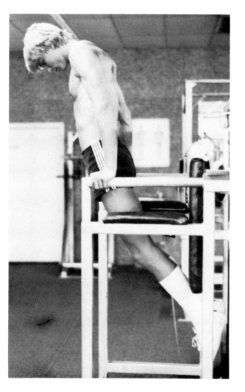 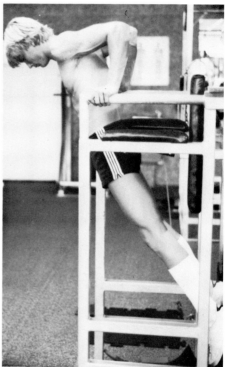

I1-2: Forward Dip

Lean forward and proceed to
press yourself upward while
maintaining the forward lean.
This will add bulk to the whole
upper body, but especially the
lower chest. You may use a
dumbbell to weigh yourself
down.

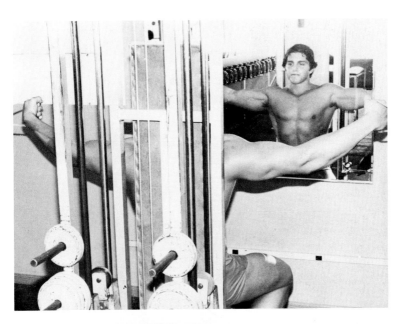

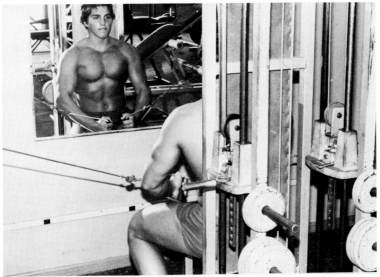

J1-3: Cable Fly

You should be seated with your
hands holding a cable and
stretched out as far as you can.
Then bring the cable almost
together in front of your chest.
This will square off your chest
and pump up your deltoids.

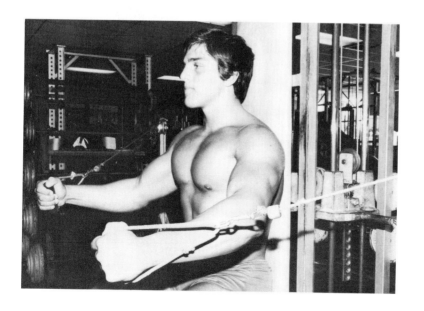

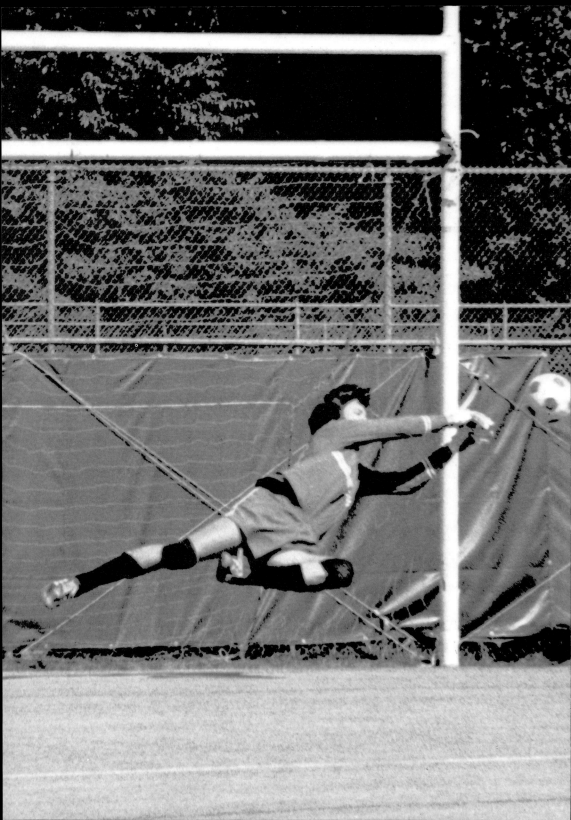

ABDOMINALS

The abdominals are comprised of abdominus rectus (that's the major part of your stomach muscles and the largest — when developed, it will look like a washerboard) the obliques (muscles on your sides — when not developed, they are commonly called *love handles*), intercoastals, and serratus magnus (a three-finger-like muscle group that lies below the rib cage). Where these muscles come together, they form a tie-in, which on a good body is very distinctive.

The most important reason for abdominal or stomach work for all athletes is to strengthen the abdominal walls in order to prevent hernias. Hernias don't just occur to football players and weight lifters but have been known to occur to baseball, basketball, and soccer players as well as to wrestlers and swimmers. Another advantage of abdominal work is that it can act as a warm-up and cool-down from your workouts. Stomach work will also help you look like an athlete, not a blob.

For those of you concerned with just general fitness or bodybuilding, developing those abs is crucial. They are crucial not just in contests but in helping a person form a positive self-image. You need to be concerned with not just the major stomach muscles but also the intercoastals, serratus and obliques.

The most important thing in getting that stomach in shape is diet. For many people that extra or wrong food such as cake, cookies, candy, ice cream, and soda appear magically at the midsection. It is crucial what you eat. Next to diet, the most important thing in developing that stomach is plenty of hard work, including running. I have met some people who have a naturally developed stomach, but they are in a very small majority. Some people use lower reps (10-25) and higher intensity exercises, such as incline sit-ups with a weight, and get great results. Others need high reps (100) on more basic exercises, such as jacknifes and partial sit-ups, to get good results. You are the only one who can tell which one works best for you. What may work for me might not work for you. Your body is like a fiddle, and you are the one best suited to play it. However, especially for the first few years of training, I recommend very basic exercises, such as incline sit-ups, leg raises, twisting, and side bends.

Watch what you eat and drink and get to work on that stomach, so you look like a champion athlete!

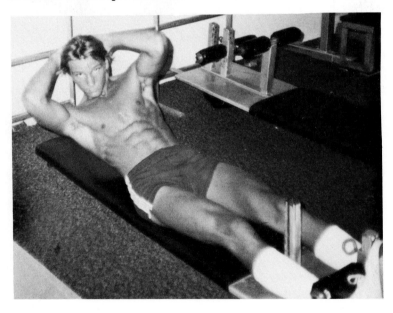

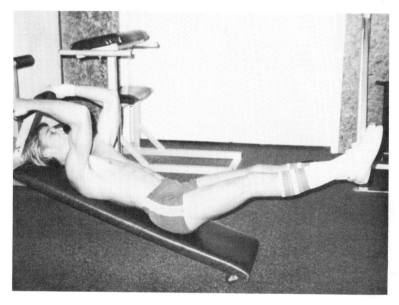

A1: Twisting Sit-Up *(left)* The twisting sit-up requires a partner to hold down your legs and is aimed at developing the oblique and abdominal muscles. Starting in a position parallel to the floor and with your hands behind your head, raise yourself, twisting as you come up from the level position three-quarters of the way up, to keep stress on your abdominals. The twist strengthens your obliques. This is also a stretching exercise utilized in warming up.

B1: Leg Raise *(above)* Raise your legs approximately 2 feet and then bring them down slowly while not touching the floor. You should do a minimum of 50 raises without stopping.

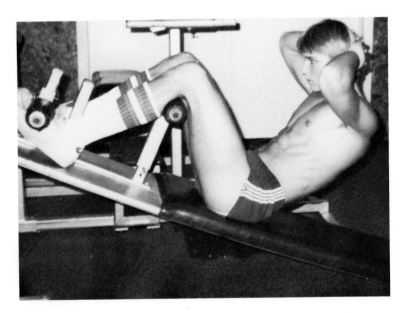

C1: Incline Sit-Up *(below)*
The inclined sit-up is performed
by bringing your knees up until
your legs are bent at a 90° angle
while your feet are in contact
with the bench or floor. Touch
your elbows to the knees while
keeping your hands together
behind your head.

D1: Wall Sit-Up *(right)*
With your legs completely
touching the wall (from the butt
up) and your hands behind your
head, try to raise up as far as you
can without moving your legs
away from the wall. This is a
very advanced exercise.

E1: Hanging Frog

Hang straight down from the bar using a shoulder-width grip. Attempt to bring your knees to your chest, but don't be disappointed if you can't do it completely. It will probably take you a few weeks before you can bring the knees all the way up to the chest.

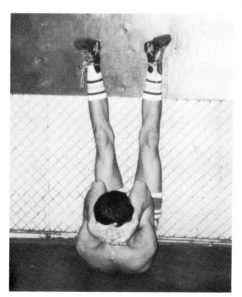

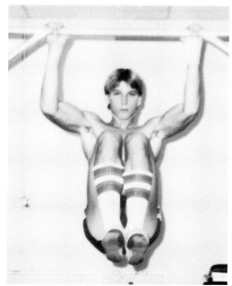

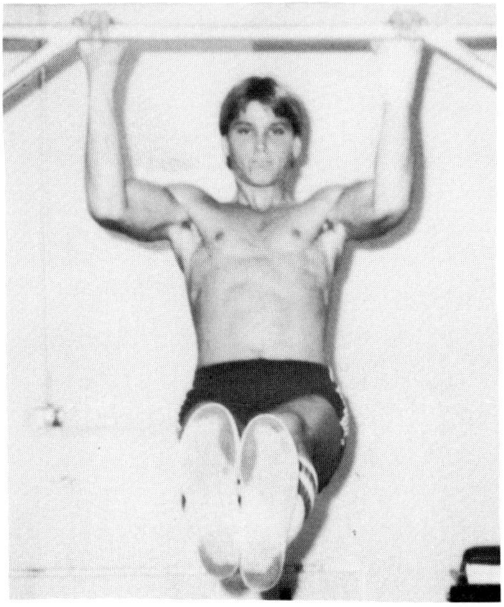

F1: Hanging Leg Raise
Hang from the bar with your legs together, and then bring your legs to a parallel position with the ground. Try to keep your legs perfectly straight.

G1-2: Jack Knife
The jack knife is a combination of a sit-up and a leg raise. With your arms outstretched and your legs kept stiff, raise your back and legs so that your hands touch your ankles.

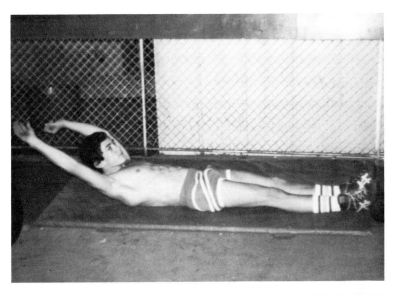

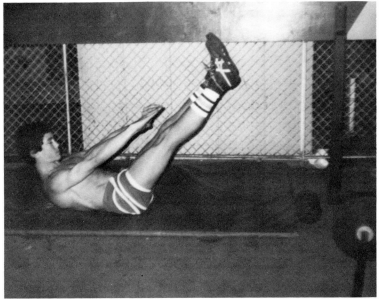

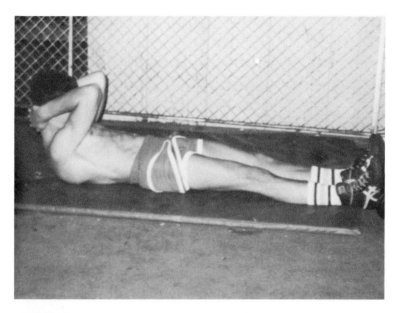

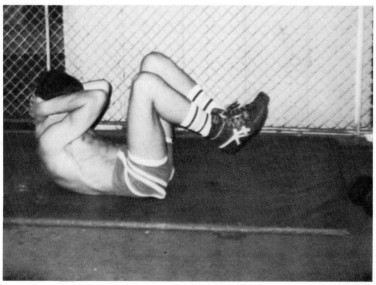

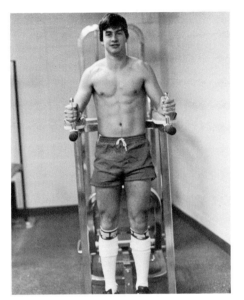 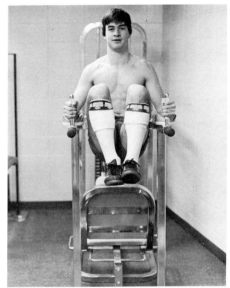

I1-2: Knee Raise
Rest your elbows on the pads
and simply pull your knees up,
bending your legs as you
proceed. Try to bring your knees
to your chest.

H1-2: Lying Knee Raise *(left)*
Fred Everts is shown performing
this exercise, which greatly
works your lower abdominals. Lie
on your back with your hands
behind your neck, and bring
your knees up toward your chest
while bending your legs.

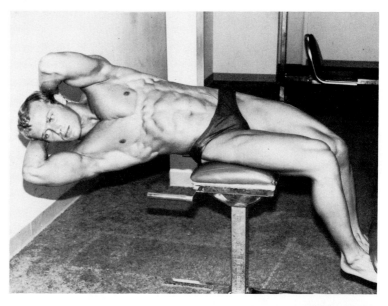

J1-2: Roman Chair Angle Sit-Up

Lie face up on the Roman chair. Then raise up from the bottom position to the top at an angle, twisting as you go up. In addition to working your abdominals, you will also work your obliques.

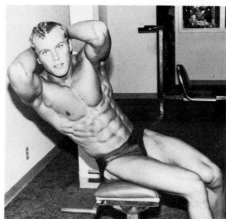

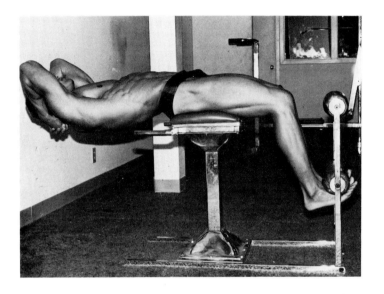

K1-2: Roman Chair Sit-Up

With your body in this same position, sit up on the Roman chair with your hands behind your neck. Slowly extend yourself backwards until you are almost touching the floor. Then raise yourself up to the seated position. This exercise will also work your lower back.

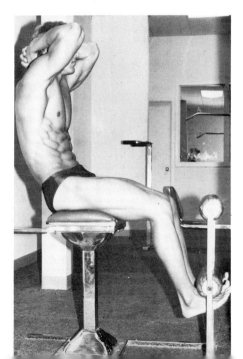

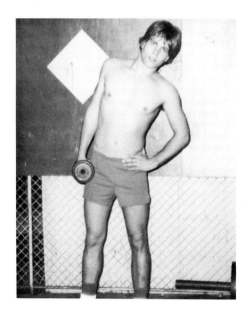

L1: Side Bend

Use a light dumbbell — 10 pounds or less — to work the oblique muscle group. Bend to the opposite side of the weight a minimum of 50 times a side. Don't use too heavy a weight, or you'll bulk the muscle more than you want to.

M1-2: Stretching and Flexing

This exercise has many different purposes. It can be used to warm up, get the blood flowing, and loosen up the back and stomach. Hold the bar behind your head and twist from side to side. It will tighten up the abdominals and obliques. Do about 150 of these twists to warm up properly.

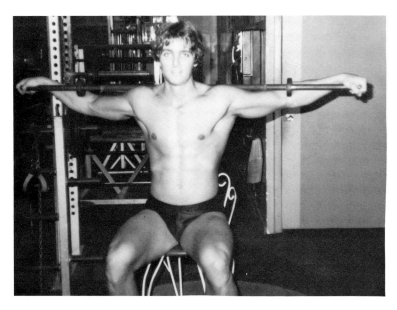

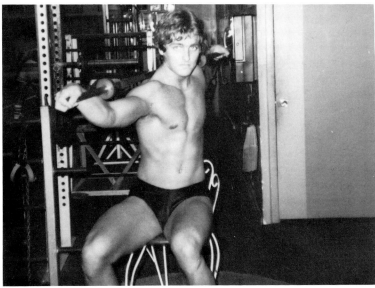

PART II:

WEIGHT PROGRAMS

BY SPORT

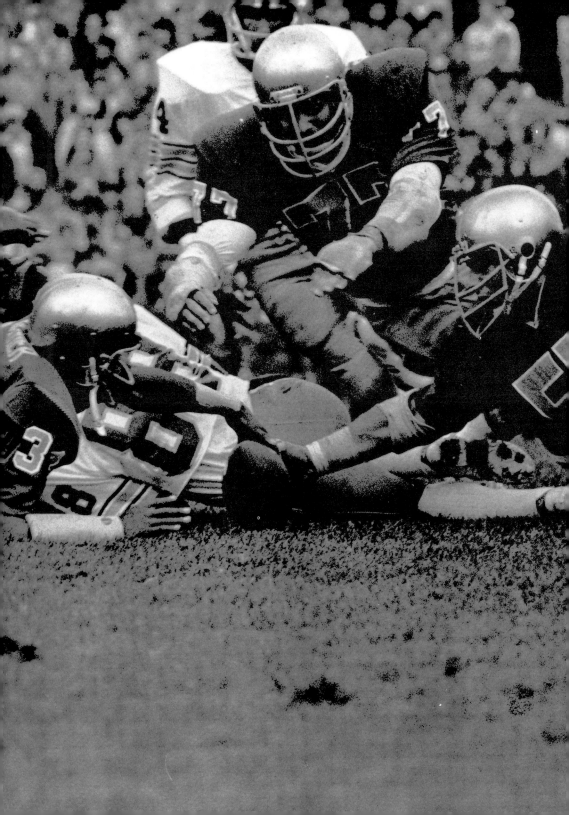

FOOTBALL

High school, college, and pro teams have been using weight training more and more, realizing that it's the one chief way to train for fewer injuries and stronger and faster players. A major reason for weight training for football teams is to keep up with other teams. Cincinnati Moeller High School in Ohio has been doing it for years and their great former coach, Gerry Faust (now head coach at Notre Dame), attributes part of their success to their weight-training program. George Smith at St. Thomas Aquinas High School in Ft. Lauderdale states that before they had an effective weight program they had lots of injuries and very seldom saw a winning team. Recently they have been consistent champions and have had their players go on to major football powerhouses such as Notre Dame and Michigan. There is virtually no professional football team that doesn't have some kind of weight program, and they even give strength tests to all men they are considering hiring.

These programs are meant to be for beginners and young football programs. If you can follow them three times a week in the off-season and maintain your strength twice a week during the season, you will be bigger, faster, stronger, and be able to play football better.

Football Programs
(Beginning football players, all positions, for the first 2 years.)

Warm-up: stretching and flexing **(Abdominals M).**

*1. 3 sets of squats **(Legs F):** 1st set for 12 reps.; 2d set for 10 reps.; 3d set for 8 reps.
*2. 3 sets of military presses **(Deltoids F):** 1st set for 12 reps.; 2d set for 10 reps.; 3d set for 8 reps.
*3. 3 sets of chin-ups **(Back M),** 12-15 reps.
 4. 3 sets of dumbbell incline curls **(Arms & Wrists I),** 12 reps.

Cool-down: 25 sit-ups, 25 leg raises **(Abdominals B),** stretching and flexing **(Abdominals M).**

(Advanced football players, after 2 years of lifting.)

Linemen

Warm-up: stretching and flexing **(Abdominals M).**

 1. 1 set of leg extensions **(Legs A),** 12 reps.
 2. 1 set of leg curls **(Legs B),** 12 reps.
*3. 5 sets of squats **(Legs F):** lst set for 12 reps; 2d set for 10 reps.; 3d set for 8 reps.; 4th and 5th sets for 6 reps.
 4. 3 sets of donkey toe raises **(Legs M),** 10 burning reps.
*5. 3 sets of dumbbell incline presses **(Chest C):** 1st set for 12 reps.; 2d set for 10 reps.; 3d set for 8 reps.
 6. 3 sets of pullovers **(Chest E),** 12 reps.
*7. 3 sets of upright rows **(Back L),** 12 reps.
*8. 3 sets of dumbbell cleans and presses **(Back M),** 8 reps.
*9. 3 sets of bent-over parallel rows **(Back A),** 12 reps.
 10. *Defensive linemen,* do lunge curls **(Arms & Wrists T);** *offensive linemen,* do dumbbell incline curls **(Arms & Wrists I).**

11. Neck machine **(Neck E or F)**, 30 seconds or 12 reps. in each position.

Cool-down: 50 sit-ups, 50 leg raises **(Abdominals B)**, stretching and flexing **(Abdominals M)**.

Linebackers & Defensive Backs

Warm-up: stretching and flexing **(Abdominals M)**.

1. 1 set of leg extensions **(Legs A)**, 12 reps.
2. 1 set of leg curls **(Legs B)**, 12 reps.
*3. 5 sets of squats **(Legs F)**: 1st set for 12 reps.; 2d set for 10 reps., 3d through 5th set for 8 reps.
4. 3 sets of donkey toe raises **(Legs M)**, 10 burning reps.
*5. 3 sets of dumbbell incline presses **(Chest C)**: 1st set for 12 reps.; 2d set for 10 reps; 3d set for 8 reps.
6. 3 sets of pullovers **(Chest E)**, 12 reps.
*7. 3 sets of upright rows **(Back L)**, 12 reps.
*8. 8 sets of dumbbell cleans and presses **(Back M)**, 8 reps.
*9. 2 sets of chin-ups **(Back M)**, 15 reps.
10. 2 sets of dumbbell rows **(Back G)**, 12 reps.
11. 3 sets of dumbbell reverse curls **(Arms & Wrists R)**, 8 reps.
12. 2 sets of wrist curls **(Arms & Wrists O & P)**: 1st set up for 20 reps.; 2d set down for 20 reps.
13. Neck machine **(Neck E or F)**, 30 seconds or 12 reps. in each position.

Cool down: 50 sit-ups and 50 leg raises **(Abdominals B)**, stretching and flexing **(Abdominals M)**.

Offensive Backs

Warm-up: stretching and flexing **(Abdominals M).**

1. 1 set of leg extensions **(Legs A)**, 12 reps.
2. 1 set of leg curls **(Legs B)**, 12 reps.
*3. 5 sets of squats **(Legs F)**, 12 reps.
4. 3 sets of donkey toe raises **(Legs M)**, 10 burning reps.
*5. *Quarterbacks:* 3 sets of close-grip bench presses **(Arms & Wrists E)**, 12 reps. *Other offensive backs:* 3 sets of dumbbell incline presses **(Chest C)**, 12 reps.
*6. 3 sets of upright rows **(Back L)**, 12 reps.
7. 3 sets of pullovers **(Chest E)**, 12 reps.
*8. 3 sets of dumbbell cleans and presses **(Back M)**, 12 reps.
9. 3 sets of chin-ups **(Back F)**, 12 reps.
10. 3 sets of dumbbell curls (any in **Arms & Wrists** section), 12 reps.
*11. 3 sets of straight dips **(Arms & Wrists G)**, as many reps as you can do.
12. Neck machine **(Neck E or F)**, 30 seconds or 12 reps. in each position.

Cool down: 50 sit-ups and 50 leg raises **(Abdominals B)**, stretching and flexing **(Abdominals M).**

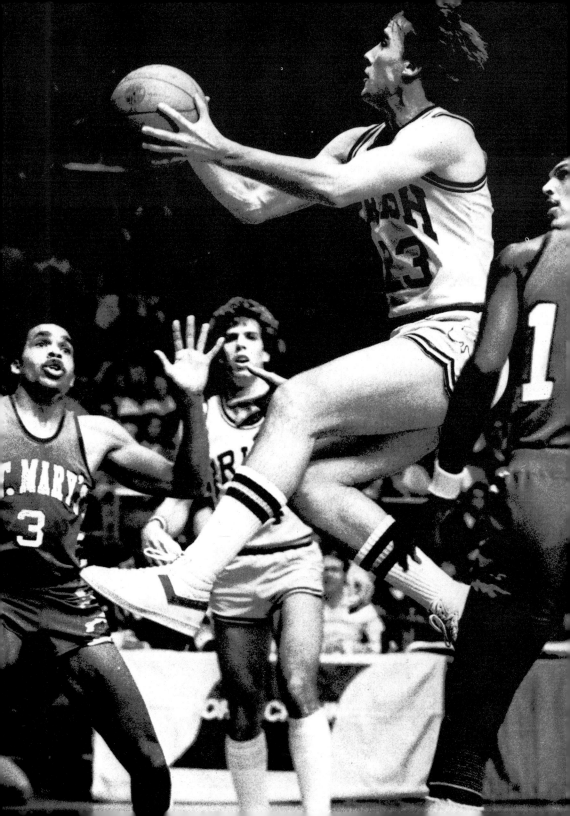

BASKETBALL

Does Adrian Dantley look inflexible? How about Kelly Tripucka of Notre Dame, or the University of Kentucky basketball team? Well, they are avid weight lifters. They believe it increases their speed, strength under the boards, jumping ability, and helps to prevent injuries. Remember also that your shoulders need to be strong to keep your arms up in defense, and your arms must be strong to hold onto the ball.

These programs are very basic, but they can help you to do all these things and be a better basketball player.

Basketball Programs
(Beginning basketball players, all positions, for the first 2 years.)

Warm-up: stretching and flexing **(Abdominals M).**
*1. 3 sets of squats **(Legs F),** 12 reps.
 2. 3 sets of step ups **(Legs K),** 12 reps.
*3. 3 sets of military presses **(Deltoids F),** 12 reps.
*4. 3 sets of underhand chin-ups **(Back O)** for as many reps. as you can do

Cool-down: 25 sit-ups and 25 legs raises **(Abdominals B),** stretching and flexing **Abdominals M).**

(Advanced basketball players, after 2 years of lifting.)

Warm-up: stretching and flexing **(Abdominals M).**
 1. 1 set of leg extensions **(Legs A),** 12 reps.
 2. 1 set of leg curls **(Legs B),** 12 reps.
*3. 5 sets of squats **(Legs F),** 12 reps.
 4. 3 sets of step ups **(Legs K),** 12 reps.
*5. 3 sets of dumbbell incline flies **(Chest F),** 12 reps.
 6. 3 sets of pullovers **(Chest E),** 12 reps.
*7. 3 sets of military presses **(Deltoids F),** 12 reps.
*8. 3 sets of chin-ups **(Back M),** as many reps. as you can do.
 9. 3 sets of dumbbell incline curls **(Arms & Wrists I),** 12 reps.
10. 2 sets of hyperextensions **(Back C),** 25 reps.

Cool-down: 50 sit-ups and 50 leg raises **(Abdominals B),** stretching and flexing **(Abdominals M).**

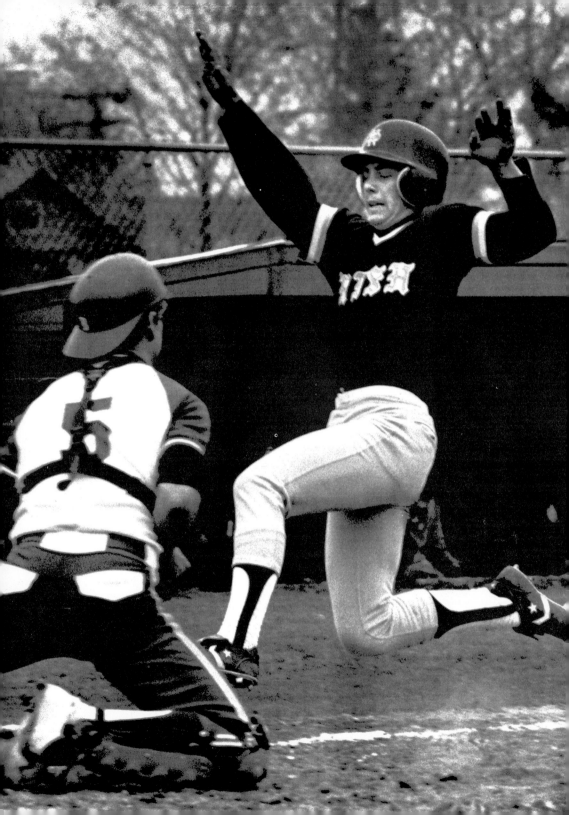

BASEBALL

One of the reasons that Carl Yastrzemski was able to play in the pros so long was his condition, which included weight training. Baseball is not just played during the season but is prepared for throughout most of the year.

After I instituted the first weight-training program for baseball at Notre Dame, the team went from a very mediocre one to a championship team that recorded the most wins ever by a Notre Dame team. Weight training could be the difference to your playing.

Baseball Programs
(Beginning baseball players, for the first 2 years.)

Warm-up: stretching and flexing **(Abdominals M).**

*1. *Pitchers and catchers:* 3 sets of squats **(Legs F),** 12 reps. *Others* may substitute 3 sets of leg presses **(Legs),** 12 reps.
  2. 3 sets of close-grip bench presses **(Arms & Wrists E),** 12 reps.
*3. 3 sets of military presses **(Deltoids F),** 12 reps.
*4. 3 sets of chin-ups **(Back M),** for as many reps as you can do.

Cool-down: 25 sit-ups and 25 leg raises **(Abdominals B),** stretching and flexing **(Abdominals M).**

(Advanced baseball players, after 2 years of lifting.)

Warm-up: stretching and flexing **(Abdominals M).**
  1. 1 set of leg extensions **(Legs A),** 12 reps.
  2. 1 set of leg curls **(Legs B),** 12 reps.
*3. *Pitchers and catchers:* 5 sets of squats **(Legs F),** 12 reps. *Others* may substitute 5 sets of leg presses **(Legs D),** 12 reps.

4. 3 sets of donkey toe raises **(Legs M)**, 10 burning reps.
*5. 3 sets of dumbbell incline presses **(Chest C)**, 12 reps.
6. 3 sets of close-grip bench presses **(Arms & Wrists E)**, 12 reps.
7. 3 sets of pullovers **(Chest E)**, 12 reps.
*8. 3 sets of chin-ups **(Back M)**, for as many reps as you can do. *Pitchers and catchers* should add 3 sets of lat pulldowns **(Back K)**, 12 reps.
*9. 3 sets of military presses **(Deltoids F)**, 12 reps.
10. *Pitchers:* 2 sets of pronating curls **(Arms & Wrists N)**, 12 reps, and 2 sets of supinating curls **(Arms & Wrists M)**, 12 reps. *Others* may do 3 sets of any kind of dumbbell curls for 12 reps.
11. 1 set of wrist curls with dumbbells up and down **(Arms & Wrists O & P)**, sideways **(Arms & Wrists S)**, and flip flops **(Arms & Wrists R)**, 20 reps. each.

Cool-down: 50 sit-ups and 50 leg raises **(Abdominals B)**, stretching and flexing **(Abdominals M)**.

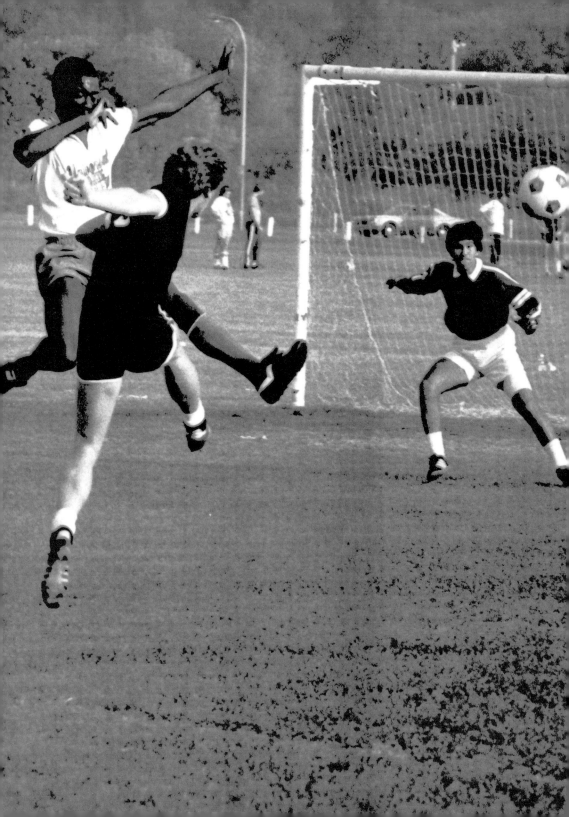

SOCCER

When I was strength coach at Notre Dame, a number of soccer players were sent to me for their secondary stage of rehabilitation by the trainer. After Coach Rich Hunter and I instituted a required weight program for soccer at Notre Dame, the number of injuries was signficantly reduced. Eighty percent of the support for your knees comes from your hams and quads; when you build these up, you significantly reduce the chance of a serious knee injury.

You are not going to go from a 5-second to a 4-second 40-yard dash, but you can improve your speed by a couple of tenths of a second by strengthening your legs through weight training. And this has been proven by hundreds of coaches around the country. I don't have to stress to you how important it is for you to be able to run faster and to have the stamina to be able to keep on running. Soccer is played on your legs. Running faster longer and kicking better requires stronger legs.

These are very basic programs but ones that will help you play with fewer injuries, run faster and longer, and kick harder. For your own sake and your team's sake, get going and start lifting!

Soccer Programs
(Beginning soccer players for the first 2 years.)

Warm-up: stretching and flexing **(Abdominals M).**

*1. 3 sets of squats **(Legs F)**, 12 reps.
*2. 3 sets of military presses **(Deltoids F)**, 12 reps.
 3. 3 sets of pullovers **(Chest E)**, 12 reps.
*4. 3 sets of underhand chin-ups **(Back O)**, 12 reps.
 5. Neck machine **(Neck E or F)**, 1 set in each position or substitute other neck exercises.

Cool-down: 25 sit-ups and 25 leg raises **(Abdominals B)**, stretching and flexing **(Abdominals M).**

(Advanced soccer players, after 2 years of lifting.)

Warm-up: stretching and flexing **(Abdominals M).**

 1. 1 set of leg extensions **(Legs A)**, 12 reps.
 2. 1 set of leg curls **(Legs B)**, 12 reps.
*3. 5 sets of squats **(Legs F)**: 1st set for 12 reps., 2d set for 10 reps., 3d through 5th set for 8 reps.
 4. 2 sets of lunges **(Legs J)**, 12 reps.
 5. 3 sets of donkey toe raises **(Legs M)**, 10 burning reps.
*6. 5 sets of bench presses **(Chest A)**: 1st set for 12 reps., 2d set for 10 reps, 3d through 5th set for 8 reps.
 7. 3 sets of pullovers **(Chest E)**, 12 reps.
*8. 3 sets of dumbbell cleans and presses **(Back M)**, 12 reps.
*9. 3 sets of back-grip chin-ups **(Back N)**, or lat pulldowns **(Back K)**, 12 reps.

10. 3 sets of curls (any kind in **Arms & Wrists** section), 12 reps.
11. 3 sets of straight dips **(Arms & Wrists G),** as many reps as you can do.
*12. Neck machine **(Neck E or F),** 30 seconds or 12 reps. in each position or substitute other neck exercise.

Cool-down: 50 sit-ups and 50 leg raises **(Abdominals B),** stretching and flexing **(Abdominals M).**

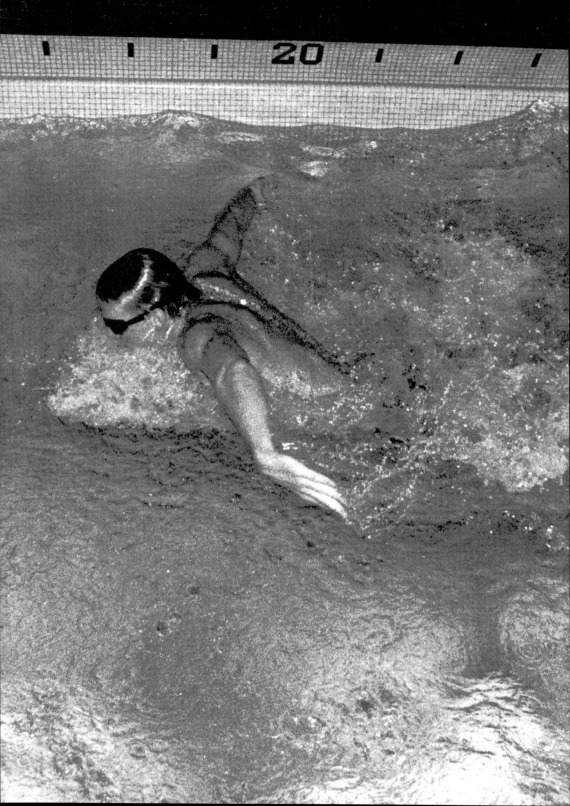

SWIMMING

Rumor had it that swimming elongates muscles while weight lifting contracts them, and that therefore the two are incompatible. Weight lifting does contract and build muscles, but even though swimming appears to be a long stretching of the muscles, which some call elongating the muscles, it also is building muscles.

You only have to look at most swimmers' chests to see how they are building their muscles through swimming. Swimmers have some of the best-developed chests of any athletes. These pectorals or chest muscles aren't developed by the breaststroke only but in all swimming motions.

Swimming is one of the most grueling of sports. You burn up to 400 calories per half hour of swimming. Swimmers are some of the most dedicated of athletes, practicing hours a day and using every muscle group in the body. That is why I recommend total-body workouts for swimmers when they are not in competition. Whether the event is the breaststroke, backstroke, free style, or a medley, all the muscles need to be built up both to help swim faster and to promote endurance.

Obviously, practicing swimming is the best way to improve, but next to that, weight training is the best thing you can do to aid your swimming. Just think about those aching pectorals, shoulders, arms, and legs after a hard practice, and you will appreciate the benefits of strengthening those muscle groups. Don't forget those legs. Leg strength, including calves, is crucial in your kicking.

Evidence that weight training is an important aid to swimmers is that most universities have weight programs included in their conditioning for swimmers. In the forefront of universities noted for their swimming teams is the University of Indiana, which has been requiring weight training of their swimmers for years. If you have the desire to swim faster and have better endurance, make sure you are following the example of champions and including weight training in your conditioning regimen.

Swimming Programs
(Beginning swimmers, for the first 2 years.)

Warm-up: stretching and flexing **(Abdominals M).**

*1. 3 sets of squats **(Legs F),** 12 reps.
 2. 3 sets of pullovers **(Chest E),** 12 reps.
*3. 3 sets of chin-ups **(Back M),** 12 reps.
*4. 3 sets of military presses **(Deltoids F),** 12 reps.

Cool-down: 50 sit-ups and 50 leg raises **(Abdominals B).**

(Advanced swimmers, after 2 years of lifting.)

Warm-up: stretching and flexing **(Abdominals M).**

 1. 1 set of leg extensions **(Legs A),** 12 reps.
 2. 1 set of leg curls **(Legs B),** 12 reps.
*3. 5 sets of squats **(Legs F):** 1st set for 12 reps.; 2d set for 10 reps.; 3d through 5th set for 8 reps.
 4. 3 sets of donkey toe raises **(Legs M),** 10 burning reps.
*5. 3 sets of lying crossover flies **(Chest H),** 12 reps.
*6. 3 sets of pullovers **(Chest E),** 12 reps.
 7. 3 sets of lat pulldowns **(Back K),** 12 reps.

*8. 3 sets of military presses **(Deltoids F),** 12 reps.
 9. 3 sets of dumbbell curls **(Arms & Wrists H),** 12 reps.
10. 3 sets of forward dips **(Chest I),** 20 reps.
11. 2 sets of hyperextensions **(Back C),** 25 reps.

Cool-down: 100 sit-ups, 100 leg raises **(Abdominals B),** 100 side bends **(Abdominals L).**

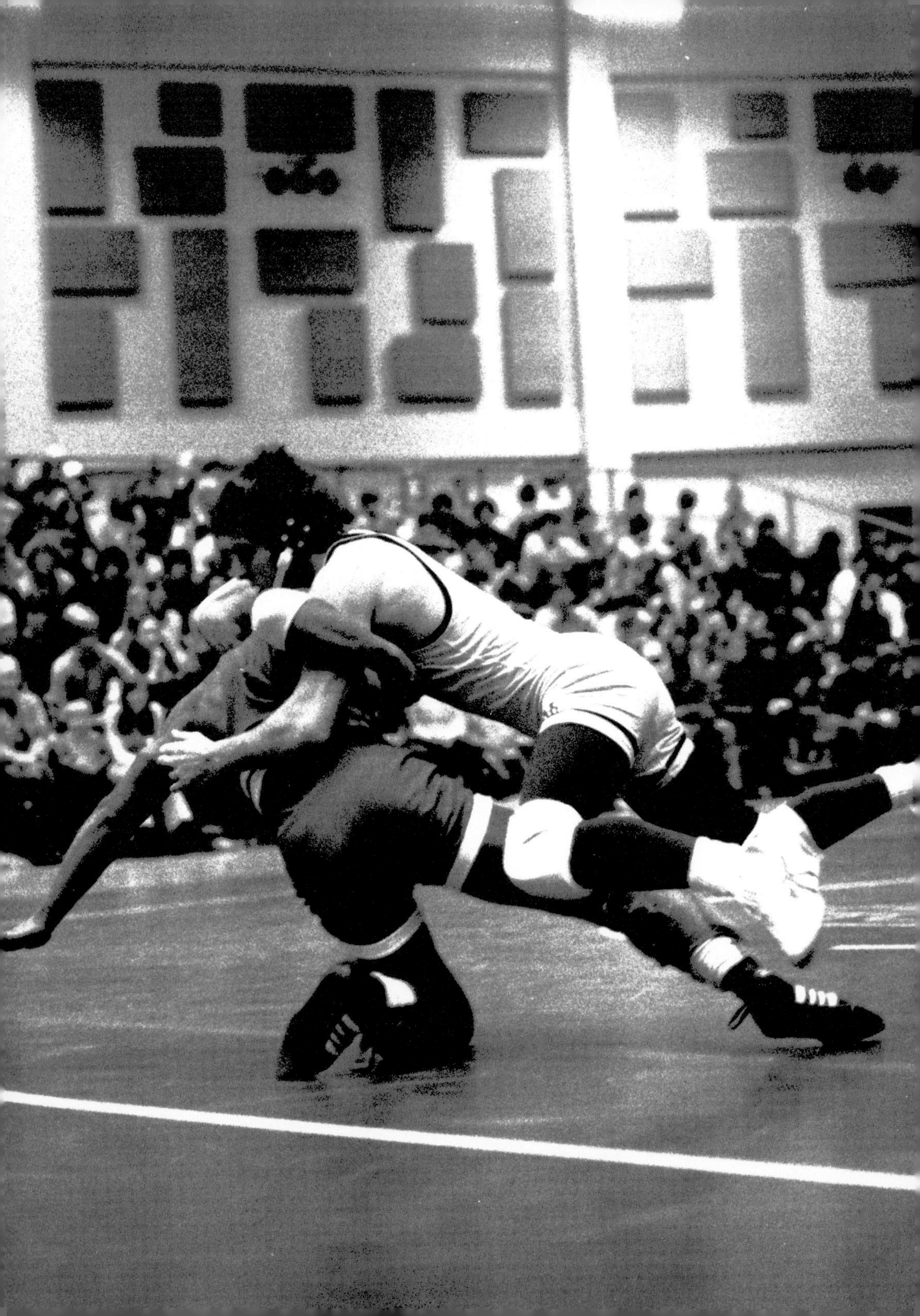

WRESTLING

Wrestling takes a lot of skill. It's one-on-one with no one there to help you, so you have to do everything you can when you are off the mat to give yourself the tools to win. Weight training for the wrestler is critical. Strength is everything in wrestling. And again you need the speed that weight training can help develop.

Shoulder injuries are fairly common in wrestling. Your shoulder is more dependent on the supporting muscle groups than any other joint. By building up those deltoids and traps, you can help to prevent that painful and incapacitating injury.

There is hardly a wrestling team in the college ranks that doesn't have a weight program. In fact, wrestling coaches have led the way in requiring and teaching weight training, they have known the importance of it for many years.

Wrestling Programs
(Beginning wrestlers, for the first 2 years.)

Warm-up: stretching and flexing **(Abdominals M)**.

*1. 3 sets of squats **(Legs F)**, 12 reps.
 2. 3 sets of dumbbell incline presses **(Chest C)**, 12 reps.
*3. 3 sets of underhand chin-ups **(Back O)**, 15 reps. or
    more.
*4. 3 sets of military presses **(Deltoids F)**, 12 reps.
*5. Neck machine **(Neck E or F)**, 30 seconds or 12 reps. in
    each position or substitute other neck exercise.

Cool-down: 25 sit ups and 25 leg raises **(Abdominals B)**,
stretching and flexing **(Abdominals M)**.

(Advanced wrestlers, after 2 years of lifting.)

Warm up: stretching and flexing **(Abdominals M)**.

 1. 1 set of leg extensions **(Legs A)**, 2 reps.
 2. 1 set of leg curls **(Legs B)**, 12 reps.
*3. 5 sets of squats **(Legs F)**: 1st set for 12 reps.; 2d set for 10
    reps.; 3d through 5th set for 8 reps.
 4. 5 sets of bench presses **(Chest A)**: 1st set for 50 percent
    of maximum for 12 reps.; 2d set 67 percent of maximum
    for 10 reps.; 3d through 5th set 82½ percent maximum
    for 4 reps.
*5. 3 sets of dumbbell incline presses **(Chest C)**, 8 reps.
 6. 3 sets of pullovers **(Chest E)**, 12 reps.
*7. 3 sets of upright rows **(Back O)**, 12 reps.
*8. 3 sets of dumbbell cleans and presses **(Back M),** 8 reps.
*9. 3 sets of T-bar rows **(Back I)**, 12 reps.
 10. 2 sets of hyperextensions **(Back C),** or good mornings
    (Back D), 20 reps.

11. 3 sets of dumbbell curls **(Arms & Wrists H),** 8 reps.
12. 2 sets of wrist curls **(Arms & Wrists O & P):** 1st set 20 reps up; 2d set 20 reps down.
*13. Neck machine **(Neck E or F),** 30 seconds or 12 reps. in each position or substitute neck other exercise.

Cool-down: 100 sit-ups and 100 leg raises **(Abdominals B),** stretching and flexing **(Abdominals M).**

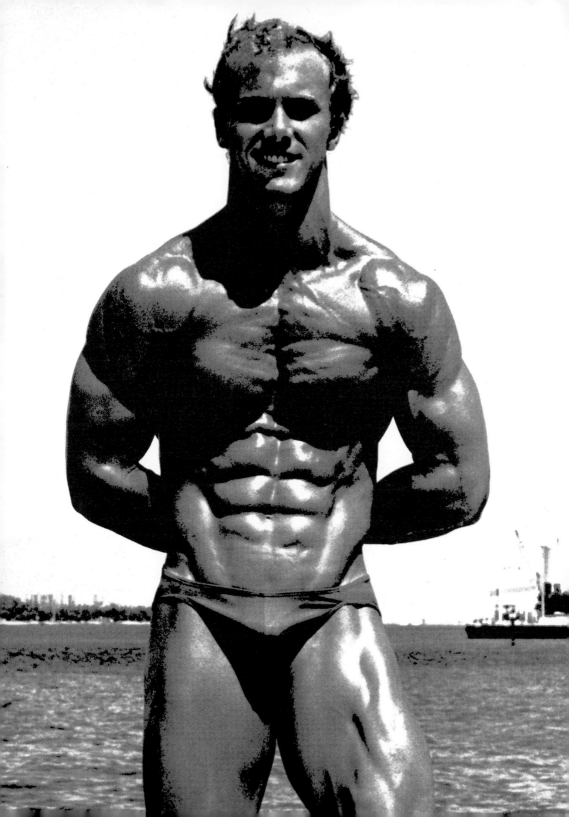

BODYBUILDING

Although Arnold Schwarzenegger and the media have helped to make most people aware of bodybuilding and to popularize it, it is not a phenomenon of the twentieth century. The ancient Greeks said that the body is the temple of the mind. If you have every seen any of their statues, you realize how they idolized "godlike" bodies. Throughout the centuries, cultures have been worshiping the body. Look at pictures of Michelangelo's David in Florence or modern-day pictures or statues of athletes.

Bodybuilding is both an art and a sport. It is a sport because you are obviously lifting weight. It is most definitely an art form because the bodybuilder's physique, his finished product, is judged in competition on an aesthetic rather than an athletic basis. The finished product, his body, is just like a piece of sculpture. The guidelines used on judging bodybuilding competition are as follows: symmetry, proportion, development, definition, structure, posing, and general appearance. The days when someone could win a bodybuilding contest solely on very large muscles are over. Definition and symmetry are necessary to win.

Bodybuilding is a long and hard sport. Thousands of hours and a difficult diet are required to make it. It takes years to make a champion, but you need a strong foundation first. That is one of the many reasons I am against steroids. If you blow up so fast on drugs, you will shrink fast when you stop. And you will have to stop or you will literally kill yourself. When you are on steroids, you tend to want quick results and try to get away from building that strong foundation. The strong foundation is built through lots of time and effort, using the basic exercises and developing the major muscle groups like the legs through squats and leg presses, the shoulders through military presses, the chest through incline presses and dips, and the arms through curls and tricep extensions.

We all can't look like Arnold because of heredity and because most of us don't want to. We just want to look good. There is nothing that you can participate in that will make you look as good as weight lifting can. Remember pictures of that skinny kid on the beach with someone kicking sand in his face? Well, that might be a little exaggerated but it is basically true. If you are a skinny kid and want to build up and look good, or if you are a chubby kid and want to shape up, get right to work on these programs, get on the right diet, and get your head straight. You can look good and be in shape. You can make your friends admire you and make people want to be your friends!

Bodybuilding Programs
(Beginning bodybuilders, for the first 2 years.)

Do the following every other day, 3 times a week.

Warm-up: push-ups, stretching and flexing **(Abdominals M).**

1. 1 set of leg extensions **(Legs A),** 12 reps.
2. 1 set of leg curls **(Legs B),** 12 reps.
3. 3 sets of squats **(Legs F),** 12 reps. (avoid this if you have back or knee problems).
4. 3 sets of bench presses **(Chest A),** 12 reps.
5. 3 sets of dumbbell incline presses **(Chest C),** 8-12 reps.
6. 3 sets of back-grip chin-ups **(Back N),** or lat pulldowns **(Back K),** 12 reps.
7. 3 sets of military presses **(Deltoids F);** 1st set for 12 reps.; 2d set for 10 reps.; 3d through 5th set for 8 reps.

8. 3 sets of curls, any kind: 1st set for 12 reps.; 2d and 3d for 8 reps.

Cool-down: 25 sit-ups and 25 leg raises **(Abdominals B)**, stretching and flexing **(Abdominals M).**

(Advanced bodybuilders, after 2 years of lifting.)

Do the following exercises every other day, 3 times a week.
Warm-up: stretching and flexing **(Abdominals M).**

1. 1 set of leg extensions **(Legs A)**, 12 reps.
2. 1 set of leg curls **(Legs B),** 12 reps.
3. 5 sets of squats **(Legs F):** 1st set for 12 reps.; 2d set for 10 reps.; 3d through 5th sets for 8 reps.
4. 3 sets of donkey toe raises **(Legs M),** 10 burning reps.
5. 5 sets of bench presses **(Chest A):** 1st set for 12 reps.
6. 3 sets of dumbbell incline presses **(Chest C),** 8 reps.
7. 3 sets of pullovers **(Chest E),** 12 reps.
8. 3 sets of upright rows **(Deltoids O),** 12 reps.
9. 3 sets of military presses **(Deltoids F):** 1st set for 12 reps.; 2d set for 10 reps.; 3d set for 8 reps.
10. 3 sets of back-grip chin-ups **(Back N),** or lat pulldowns **(Back K),** 12 reps.
11. 3 sets of dumbbell incline curls **(Arms & Wrists I),** 8 reps.
12. 3 sets of straight dips **(Arms & Wrists G),** as many reps. as you can do.
13. 2 sets of hyperextensions **(Back C),** or good mornings **(Back D),** 25 reps. Avoid this if you have back problems.

Cool-down: 50 sit-ups and 50 leg raises **(Abdominals B),** stretching and flexing **(Abdominals M).**

COACH'S
CHECKLIST

1. Make sure you know each athlete's physical condition and injury record. Keep note of his physical problems, whether it be cartilage damage to the knee, chronic shoulder separation, hamstring pulls, or a proclivity toward some specific injury.

2. Make sure that you adjust the injured player's program accordingly and in conjunction with the team's physician.

3. With the aid of the team's physician, regularly test and treat the injured player's problem area.

4. Test the player's quadriceps (with leg extensions) and hams (with leg curls) before he begins practicing. Periodically recheck. The hams-to-quadriceps stretch ratio should be 2:3. That is, the hams should be two-thirds as strong as the quadriceps. When this ratio is out of proportion, such an athlete is *very* susceptible to hamstring pulls and, possibly, strains.

5. Test your player's neck strength before allowing him to practice. He should be able to use *at least* 3 plates in each position on the Nautilus Neck Machine for at least 5 repetitions. Remember to have him keep the body stiff and use only the neck, fully extending it.

6. Before embarking on any weight program, your players should do some form of calisthenics for at least a week or have weight-training experience.

7. Make sure your players have warmed up properly. A few teams require as much as 6 minutes of stretching before warming up. Although this might be excessive, stretches, sit-ups, and push-ups are quite good.

8. Watch the player's form; try to have him perform his exercises with as perfect form as possible.

PLAYER'S CHECKLIST

1. Make sure your coach, trainer, and doctor know of any physical problems or proclivities toward injury you have.
2. If you are injured, work your rehabilitation into re-arranged strength workouts.
3. Warm up properly!
4. Use strict form on your exercises. This is the only way to get the most out of them.
5. Always try to have a training partner; it helps, and it's safer.
6. Use weight-room etiquette. Be considerate.
7. Try to get that extra repetition when you have a spotter. Your muscles get used to the weight and reps. after a short while. Strive to push ahead.
8. Cool down properly. Don't forget your sit-ups, leg raises, and stretches. Try to look like an athlete—not a blob!
9. Keep a positive attitude. I will get stronger; I will pump more weight!

GLOSSARY

Bodybuilding: an art and a sport in which you build up your body's muscle size and symmetry and display it artistically at a show.

Carbs: carbohydrates.

Cold: when your muscles aren't pumped up.

Compound set: doing two sets of exercises that work the same muscle groups, such as doing a set of barbell curls immediately followed by a set of dumbbell curls.

Flexed: when you contract your muscle.

Free weights: barbells and dumbbells.

Machines: weight-training equipment, which may use pulleys, cams, cables, hydraulics, or some other mechanical device. The most common machines are Universal, Paramount, Nautilus, Kaiser Cams, and Marcy gyms.

Olympic lifting: a sport consisting of the snatch and the clean and jerk. Unlike power lifting, which is based on brute strength, these lifts take considerable athletic ability and, therefore, are much harder to perform. They are the weight-lifting part of the Olympics.

Power lifting: a sport that consists of three exercises: the squat, bench press, and the dead lift. You compete according to weight, as in wrestling.

Pumped up: when your muscles are gorged with blood from performing a hard weight-lifting exercise. Being pumped can add up to an inch to your muscle size for up to two hours.

Recuperation: the time needed to recover or get back your strength and/or size.

Rep: repetition.

Reverse grip: when you hold a bar with one hand palms up and the other hand palms down (e.g., as in a dead lift).

Ripped: when you have great muscular definition, with veins showing (also called *cut*).

Set: a series of repetitions: a number of repetitions done together.

Smooth: when your body doesn't show fine definition of muscles (and the veins are not showing).

Superset: doing two sets together that work opposing muscle groups, such as supersetting a curl, which works the biceps, and a tricep extension, which works the triceps.

Supplements: vitamins, minerals, and protein drinks.

Vascularity: when your veins are standing out clearly visible.

Weight-lifting: the athletic exercise or competitive sport of lifting barbells

YOUR PROGRAM

date					
weight					
waist					
chest					
forearm					
upper arm					
calves					
thigh					
bench press					
dumbbell incline press					
dumbbell clean & press					

INDEX

This book has been designed to allow the user to find specific exercises quickly. The right running head (top of the right-hand page) has the chapter names in boldface type. If an exercise appears on that page or the adjacent left-hand page, the exercise letter designation will appear next to the boldface name. Thus, **Deltoids A-B** at the top would indicate that the first two deltoid exercises (in this case, the front deltoid raise and the bent-over lateral raise) appear on the indicated pages. By quickly thumbing through the book, the reader can easily find the exercise he wishes. The index below, therefore, gives the chapter name and letter instead of the page numbers, as is more common in indexes.

Flip-over hamstring stretch,
Flexibility F
Forward dip, **Chest I**
Front deltoid raise, **Deltoids A**
Front squat, **Legs G**

Good morning exercise, **Back D**

Hack squat, **Legs H**
Hamstring groin stretch I,
Flexibility H
Hamstring groin stretch II,
Flexibility I
Hamstring lower-back stretch,
Flexibility K
Hamstring stretch I, **Flexibility C**
Hamstring stretch II, **Flexibility D**
Hamstring trunk rotation,
Flexibility B
Hanging frog, **Abdominals E**
Hanging leg raise, **Abdominals F**
Hurdler's stretch, **Flexibility M**
Hyperextension, **Back C**

Incline fly, **Chest F**
Incline sit-up, **Abdominals C**
Isometric neck exercise, **Neck B**

Jack knife, **Abdominals G**

Knee raise, **Abdominals I**

Lat pulldown, **Back K**
Leg curl (Nautilus), **Legs B**
Leg extension, **Flexibility O**
Leg extension, (Nautilus), **Legs A**
Leg press, **Legs D**
Leg press (Paramount), **Legs C**
Leg raise, **Abdominals B**
Lotus groin stretch, **Flexibility J**
Lunge curl, **Arms & Wrists T**
Lying crossover Fly, **Chest H**
Lying flat fly, **Chest G**
Lying knee raise, **Abdominals H**
Lying tricep extension, **Arms &
Wrists D**

Military press, *see* power clean &
military press, **Back P**; standing
military press, **Deltoids F**
Modified hurdler's stretch,
Flexibility L

Neck harness, **Neck D**
Neck machine (Hydra-Gym), **Neck
F**
Neck machine (Nautilus 4-way),
Neck E
Negative dip, **Flexibility N**

One-arm concentrated curl, **Arms
& Wrists H**

❖❖❖

Icarus Press
P.O. Box 1225
South Bend, IN 46624

Please send me the following books:

_____ copy(ies) **Shape Up for Soccer**
    ☐ clothbound ($14.95)   ☐ wirebound ($9.95)

_____ copy(ies) **The Notre Dame Weight-Training Program for Football**
    ☐ clothbound ($12.95)   ☐ wirebound ($9.95)

_____ copy(ies) **The Notre Dame Weight-Training Program for Baseball, Hockey, Wrestling, & Your Body**
    ☐clothbound ($14.95)   ☐ wirebound ($9.95)

_____
name

_____
street address

_____
city/state/zip

Indiana residents, please add 4% sales tax. (Thank you.)

☐ Payment enclosed.

☐ Please bill my ☐ VISA or ☐ Master Charge account.

Account no. _____ expiration date _____

BUSINESS REPLY LABEL
First class   Permit No. 5   Notre Dame, IN 46556

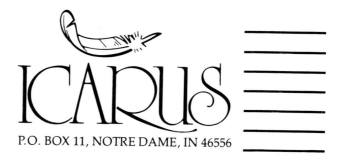

P.O. BOX 11, NOTRE DAME, IN 46556